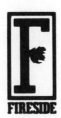

FIRESIDE

BOOKS BY Ellington Darden

Nutrition and Athletic Performance
Especially for Women
Strength-Training Principles
Olympic Athletes Ask Questions About
    Exercises and Nutrition
How to Lose Body Fat
Soccer Fitness
How Your Muscles Work
Nutrition for Athletes: Myths and Truths
Conditioning for Football
The Superfitness Handbook
The Nautilus Book: An Illustrated Guide to Physical
    Fitness the Nautilus Way
The Athlete's Guide to Sports Medicine
Power Racquetball
The Nautilus Nutrition Book

THE DARDEN TECHNIQUE

FOR

WEIGHT LOSS,
BODY SHAPING,
AND
SLENDERIZING

BY

ELLINGTON DARDEN, Ph.D.

**Photography by
Scott LeGear**

A FIRESIDE BOOK
Published by Simon and Schuster
NEW YORK

First Fireside Edition, 1982
A Fireside Book
Published by Simon & Schuster, Inc.
Simon & Schuster Building
Rockefeller Center
1230 Avenue of the Americas
New York, New York 10020

Published by arrangement with RM Marketing

FIRESIDE and colophon are registered trademarks
of Simon & Schuster, Inc.

Manufactured in the United States of America

10 9 8 7 6 5 4   Pbk.

Library of Congress Cataloging in Publication Data

Darden, Ellington, date.
   The Darden technique for weight loss, bodyshaping
and slenderizing.

   Bibliography: p.
1. Reducing exercises. I. Title.
RA781.6.D37   1982   613.7'1   81-17382
                                         AACR2
ISBN 0-671-44228-7 Pbk.

DIRECTOR OF PROJECT: Ed Shipley
PHOTOGRAPHY: Scott LeGear
ART DIRECTORS: Richard Bickhart, Susan Roberts
MODELS: Lona Dion, Ann Baker, Taca Bryan, and Ellington Darden
EDITORS: Ilanon Moon and Dale Moore
TYPESETTING: ARC Photo Comp Ltd.

CONTENTS

A Message from Jack LaLanne

I am so excited that you are about to get started reshaping your body. As you may or may not know, I have spent 50 years of my life as a Physical Culturist helping people, like you, to look better and feel better. I am sure that we are in full agreement that there is a growing obesity problem in our great country. So much has been written about it that one hardly knows where to turn and how much of the information available is valid.

The main reason I am so excited about this book is that it gives you the most modern scientific facts about weight loss and I know in my heart, if you follow the instructions and advice, you will get results far beyond your fondest hopes.

I know only too well your problems. As a boy, I was a sugarholic. I was hooked on junk foods. To break the habit, it took discipline and will power. Because of this dedication, I found it wasn't that difficult to overcome my poor eating habits. I just exchanged a few bad habits for good ones. It was that simple. Remember, you and I are the sum total of our habits. If you are fat and out of shape, you made it happen. By the same token, you have the power to correct it. The Good Book says that we are fearfully and wonderfully made. Regardless of your present age or physical condition you can change it all around, for the better.

Visualize yourself as healthy, trim, fit, and youthful. As a man thinketh, so is he. Each day that you use your discipline and will power the stronger it gets. A great philosopher once said, "Each step I take today makes the steps easier tomorrow."

The major priority in your life should be your weight-loss program. If you fall by the wayside and go off your program, don't give up! Start again!

The secret is to keep going, keep forging ahead to your goal.

My mother was a great influence in my life and lived to be 94 years young by following the principles of corrective exercise and natural foods. She was always reminding me, "Jack, anything is possible in life. Just remember, God helps them that help themselves." I know you will help yourself.

I would like to thank Dr. Darden, who is one of the top physical conditioning research experts in the country today, for his unselfish work in putting together this most comprehensive book of weight loss. I am proud to recommend such a worthy program and I know it will change many thousands of lives.

HERE'S TO A NEW YOU! MAY OUR WAISTLINES GET SMALLER AND OUR FRIENDSHIPS GET BIGGER.

Healthfully yours,

Jack LaLanne

PREFACE

By Ellington Darden, Ph.D.

Women everywhere are body conscious. Skirts with slits up the sides are in fashion. Tight, designer jeans accentuate shapely hips and thighs. The no-bra look is still popular. Jogging suits and tennis attire are as prevalent in malls and supermarkets as they are for the actual sports participation. If the fashion industry and women's magazines have their way, a slender, shapely body will always be in vogue. The designer's influence is so strong, that 90 percent of the women in the United States are dissatisfied with their figures. Every year, they spend over $40 billion on useless weight-reducing drugs, fad diet books, phoney slenderizing machines, and nonproductive exercise courses.

For the last few years, the media have been promising women sleek, slender bodies from a minimum of effort. Unfortunately, much of this media advertising is false. The science of weight reduction and body shaping has never had more to offer than it does today. Yet for every dollar that is spent publicizing scientific facts, at least a thousand dollars are used to promote fitness fraud.

The current field of weight reduction and body fitness is dominated by cultists, mystics, misinformed movie stars, hard-headed athletes, well-meaning dabblers, and outright imposters. Most of these exploiters merely want money. A few, more confused than crooked, seek converts to their ignorance.

Surveys show that in the last five years there has been a several-hundred-percent increase in the women who are participating in activities such as tennis, jogging, yoga, racquetball, calisthenics, slimnastics, aerobic dancing, and weight training.

There is no doubt that this trend will increase throughout the 1980's. More women in the United States are exercising than ever before. Yet, a trip to any beach during the summer months will convince anyone that most women are obtaining no lasting benefits from the time and effort spent on their body fitness programs. How could they when 9 out of every 10 women on the beach have flabby thighs, broad behinds, pot bellies, double chins, droopy arms, or sagging breasts?

Women are being misled and lied to about body fitness. There are no magic pills, no potions, no quick and easy remedies.

Going from fatness to fitness is among the most difficult tasks a woman can undertake. It takes self-discipline, motivation, and patience. It requires the application of scientific principles of weight reduction and body shaping. But it can be done.

Every woman in the United States who is not pleased with her figure can improve that figure. Excessive body fat can be lost permanently with the proper diet. Various parts of the body can be toned and beautified with the right kind of exercise. Proper nutrition combined with proper exercise will create a slender figure. *The Darden Technique for Weight Loss, Body Shaping and Slenderizing* was written for women who wish to achieve these goals. Hundreds of exercises are described, illustrated, and evaluated. Numerous diets are compared.

This book contains the most up-to-date, scientific information on body fitness. Women who practice the discipline demanded here will be rewarded with slender, firm, shapely figures.

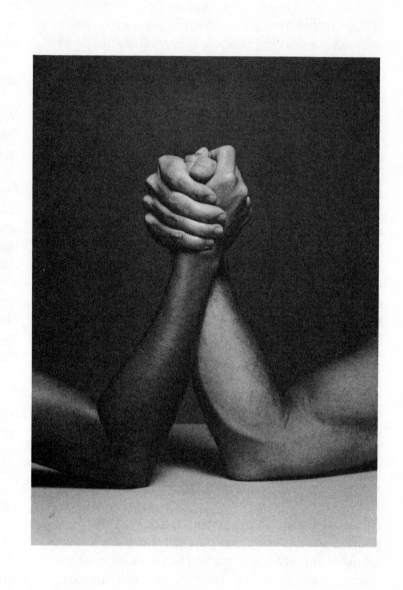

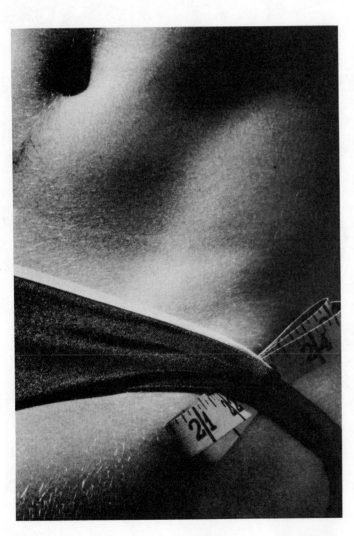 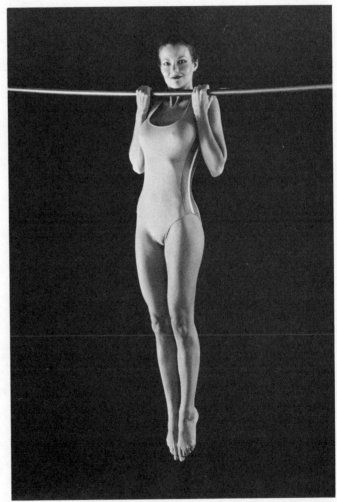

I. BASICS

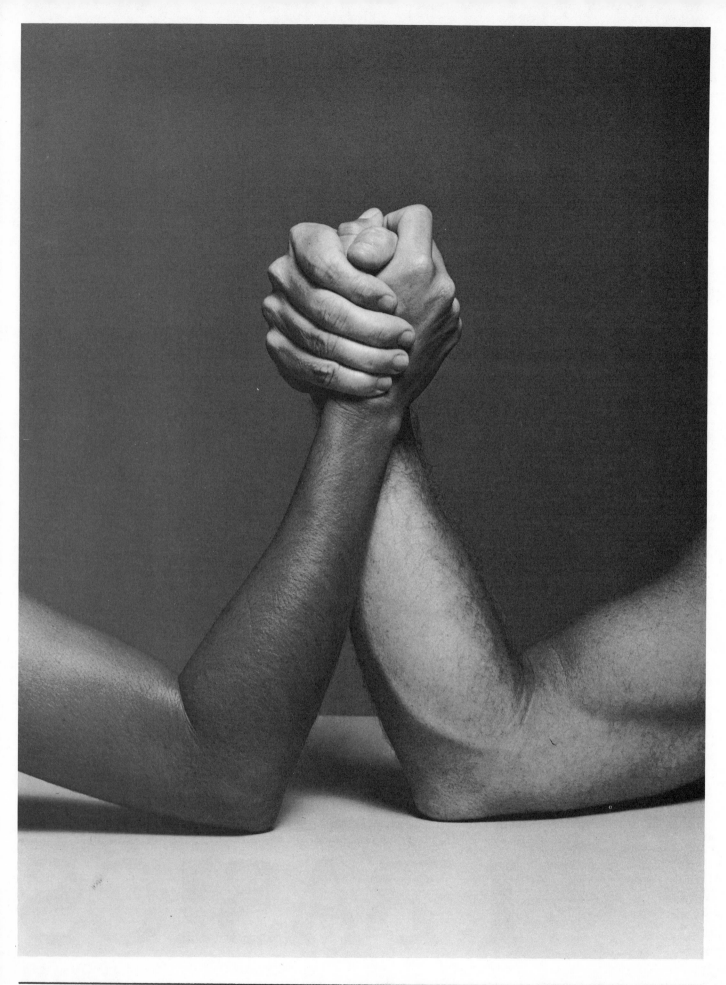

CHAPTER 1
THE TRUTH ABOUT EXERCISE

Almost every woman has opinions about exercise: how to, how not to, how much, what kind, and why. Many of these opinions come from parents, friends, teachers and coaches. Some are hand-me-down tradition. Others evolve from cleverly designed advertisements. At least three out of four of these notions are based on ignorance and false beliefs. But sound physiological facts answer the questions women ask about exercise.

Q. What is exercise?
A. The dictionary defines exercise as "...exertion of the muscles to maintain bodily health."

Exercise, however, is better defined as "movement against resistance." Without resistance, there is no effective exercise. For the body to become more shapely the muscles have to become stronger. Muscles will not become stronger unless they are taxed with an overload. Once they are overloaded, a chemical reaction takes place within the body that causes the muscles to become stronger and better proportioned.

The quality of the overload or resistance determines the value of the exercise.

According to the laws of physics, everything we do involves movement which is met by some kind of resistance. Running provides resistance. Swimming provides resistance. Jumping provides resistance. Any type of muscle-powered movement is met by some kind of resistance -- air, water, gravity or friction. Exercises using an individual's bodyweight against air, water, or gravity, however, are not very effective ways to overload the muscles. After a short time it becomes increasingly difficult to make such movements progressively more taxing.

Adding progressive resistance to the arms, legs, torso, and other parts of the body offers a much more efficient way to overload the muscles. This type of exercise has been employed in the United States for over 50 years. It is called weight training.

Weight training generally uses adjustable metal discs or weights that are loaded on bars. The long bars are called barbells, and the short ones are dumbbells. Recently, weight training has become more complex with the addition of many types of sophisticated machines. For busy women in the home, however, neither barbells nor machines are necessary. Weight training can be simplified by using common household items to furnish weight. Plastic bottles, cans, books, and other items that weigh less than 10 pounds can work surprisingly well for women.

Weight training can produce body-shaping

results impossible to obtain in any other way. This is true only because weight training provides more and better resistance. Properly applied, weight training supplies resistance where it is needed to the degree it is needed.

Millions of women are practicing worthless exercises or performing worthless exercises in such a manner that little or no resistance is offered to their muscles. Consequently, their unopposed motion has no body-shaping value.

Q. Does heavy exercise make a woman develop large muscles?

A. Most women believe if they do heavy exercises, their muscles will become large and unfeminine. But it is virtually impossible for a woman to develop large muscles.

Building large muscles requires two factors. First, the individual must have long muscle bellies and short tendon attachments. Second, an adequate amount of male hormones, particularly testosterone, must be present in the bloodstream. Women almost never have either of these factors.

Under no circumstances could 99.99 percent of American women develop large muscles. But heavy exercise is important for them because it strengthens their muscles, prevents injuries, and turns the body into trimmer and more shapely flesh.

Q. What about all those women athletes with large muscles?

A. It should be clearly understood that most women do not have the genetic potential to develop unusually large muscles. The men and women with large muscles are genetic freaks. The vast majority of women involved in Olympic and professional sports have slim, well-toned bodies. It is unfortunate that certain photographs and publicity have led people to believe that women athletes with large muscles are the rule rather than the rare exception.

During the Montreal Olympic Games, there were many very tall women playing basketball. One Russian player, Iuli Semenova, was 7 feet 2 inches tall. A teammate of hers measured 6 feet 8 inches tall. Most of the women on the medal winning teams were over 6 feet.

After watching several Olympic basketball games, a woman might assume that bouncing a ball would make her taller. She might try various ball bouncing routines with no success and conclude that bouncing a ball had no effect on increasing her height. She might also realize that if she grew in height it would be her genetic inheritance and not her ball-bouncing.

The same is true for the very few women with large muscles. They have inherited above-average length muscles and above-average levels of male hormones. They have the ability to develop larger and more defined muscles than the typical woman. These few women will be larger and stronger than the average woman even if they never exercise or take part in sports.

If a woman who had all the genetic capabilities actually did develop unsightly muscles, she could go without exercise for a week and her muscles would shrink. Muscles are made to be used. If they are not used, they atrophy.

Q. What is the difference between body building and body shaping?

A. Body building is basically a masculine term that is used to describe the exercises that men do with weights to strengthen and proportion their bodies. Some of these men, usually the ones with the most genetic potential, eventually compete in body building or physique contests. The winners have broad shoulders, narrow hips, long muscle bellies in their arms and legs, and little body fat.

The average man can increase his strength approximately 300 percent before he reaches his full potential. The typical woman can increase her strength about 150 percent. Since the average woman has approximately twice as much fat as the average man, muscles do not stand out on a woman as they do on a man. Women who train with weights do so to shape, tone, and beautify their bodies. The goal of resistance for women, therefore, is body shaping.

Q. Which muscles are most important for a woman?

A. Both men and women have 434 skeletal muscles. Much of the face, neck, torso, hips, legs, and arms consists of muscles. They range in size from the tiny eye to large hip muscles. All are composed of long slim fibers bound in bundles. The major muscles of the feminine figure are named on the following photographs.

Some women, depending on their particular problem areas will want to concentrate on strengthening and shaping certain muscle groups. Most women, however, should exercise all their major muscles at least twice a week. A woman should not take any of her muscles for granted.

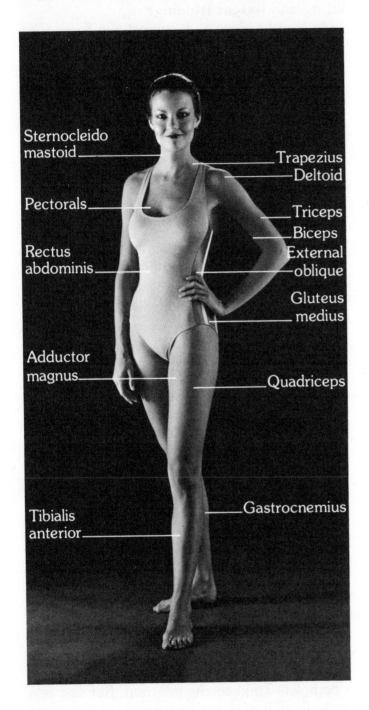

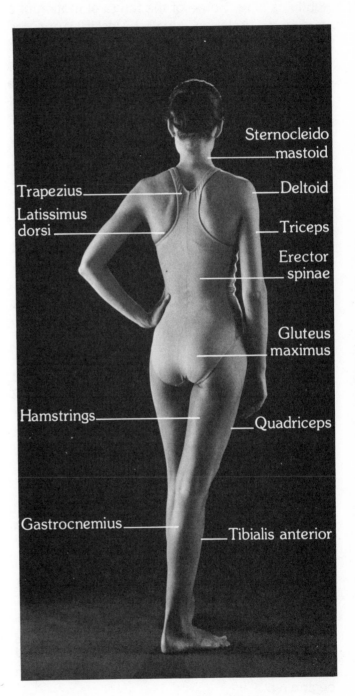

BASICS: THE TRUTH ABOUT EXERCISE

Q. Will heavy exercise make a woman tight and inflexible?

A. No. The exact opposite is true. Heavy exercise properly performed will make a woman more flexible.

Body flexibility is the ability to stretch and contract muscles throughout a full range of motion. The use-or-lose-it principle applies nowhere as cogently as here. Some of the range of motion of a particular muscle can actually be lost if it is not used throughout its full stretching and contracting process. A woman can become tight and inflexible by using her muscles too little. This can easily be observed in the stiff walk or shuffle of the elderly.

Proper body-shaping exercises apply resistance to the muscles as they are stretched and contracted. Muscles that have been trained in this manner are not only stronger but more flexible.

Q. What happens if a woman exercises and gets into good condition and then stops working out? Will her muscles turn to fat?

A. Absolutely not! Muscles are muscles, and fat is fat. There is no way a woman can turn one into the other.

Muscles are composed of 70 percent water, 22 percent proteins, and 7 percent lipids. Fat is 22 percent water, 6 percent protein, and 72 percent lipids. So like apples and oranges, muscle and fat though similar in composition, are genetically and chemically different.

When a woman stops training, she seldom decreases her caloric intake. As a result, she has a gradual decrease in the shape and strength of her muscle mass and an increase in body fat stores. Since muscle and fat are so close to each other that they can intermingle, it appears that her muscles have turned to fat. Fortunately, this does not happen immediately. She can stop exercising completely and work back to her previous level of condition in a fraction of the time it took in the beginning.

Q. Is strenuous exercise dangerous?

A. The danger in most exercise lies not in its exertion, but the speed of its movement. Any exercise performed suddenly in a fast, jerky fashion is dangerous. The very same exercise, however, can be completely safe if it is performed slowly and smoothly. Slow, smooth movement is not only the safest way to exercise. It is by far the most productive.

Q. What is the difference between weight lifting and weight training?

A. Weight lifting is a competitive sport. The goal of weight lifting is to raise as much weight on a barbell as possible while maintaining a certain form. Weight lifting not only requires strength but great skill. Anyone who has watched the Superstars competition on television can testify to that. Many big strong athletes perform poorly in weight lifting competition because they lack the skill to lift a heavy barbell over their heads.

Few people know that weight lifting is probably the most dangerous sport in existence today. Lifting, or a better word would be throwing, a heavy weight suddenly can easily damage the tendons, ligaments, and muscles that surround all the major joints. Women should never attempt weight lifting.

Weight training, however, is a very effective activity for developing the feminine form. It is not competitive, nor does it have the same goal as weight lifting. Its purpose is the strengthening and beautifying of the body. Instead of a one-time, sudden exertion, a woman lifts the weight slowly and smoothly 8 to 12 times. Perfect form and the correct number of repetitions are what really count.

Proper weight training is body shaping. It is one of the safest forms of exercise a woman can engage in. It is certainly the most effective way to strengthen, tone, and slenderize her body.

Q. Is running the best overall exercise for women?

A. No. Weight training is much better. It can be a complete conditioning program. Running is a limited, midrange activity involving the large muscles of the lower half of the body. Although running can develop high levels of heart-lung endurance, it can actually reduce overall levels of muscular strength and flexibility. Running can also cause joint damage from excessive jarring every time the woman's foot hits the ground.

Q. Can body-shaping exercise be done at home?

A. Yes. Most of the exercises described in this book are designed for use in the home. Some exercises can be performed with bodyweight alone. Others require the use of chairs, books, cans, and plastic bottles filled with water. Barbells and dumbbells, if available, can provide even better results.

Women who have access to Nautilus exercise machines should most definitely use them. Nautilus machines provide the most efficient way for a woman to shape and strengthen her body.

Q. Exactly what are Nautilus machines?

A. Nautilus machines are scientifically designed around the physics of the human body. With their unique system of chains, sprockets, cams, and weights, they provide full-range exercise for all the major muscle groups. Nautilus machines are usually found in fitness centers, health clubs, and university training rooms. Chapter 17 provides instruction on how to use the Nautilus machines for best results.

Q. Will certain body-shaping exercising make a woman sore?

A. Almost any type of unusual muscular activity will cause temporary soreness in even the best-conditioned athletes. Women should not let a little soreness discourage their body-shaping program. To ease the soreness, a woman should repeat the same exercises that made her sore . After the first week of exercising, the soreness is not likely to return.

Q. Can a woman be too old for body-shaping exercises?

A. No one is ever too old to start a body-shaping program. Any woman with diabetes, high blood pressure, or a history of cardiovascular problems, however, should consult her personal physician before beginning an exercise program.

Since many older women are inactive, they often lose much of their muscular shape, tone, strength, and flexibility. Weight-training and body-shaping exercises provide an excellent way to improve these important factors in a systematic, progressive procedure.

Q. Should a woman exercise during her period?

A. For many years, there has been a prevalent misconception that women should exert themselves as little as possible during their periods. Current medical research indicates that all phases of menstrual difficulties from premenstrual tension to menstrual cramps are eased or even eliminated with proper exercise.

Q. Is weight training a good way to condition the body for sports?

A. Yes, indeed. Movement in sport is a result of muscular contraction. Keeping the muscles strong and in prime condition will help a woman perform any sport better and with a reduced probability of injury.

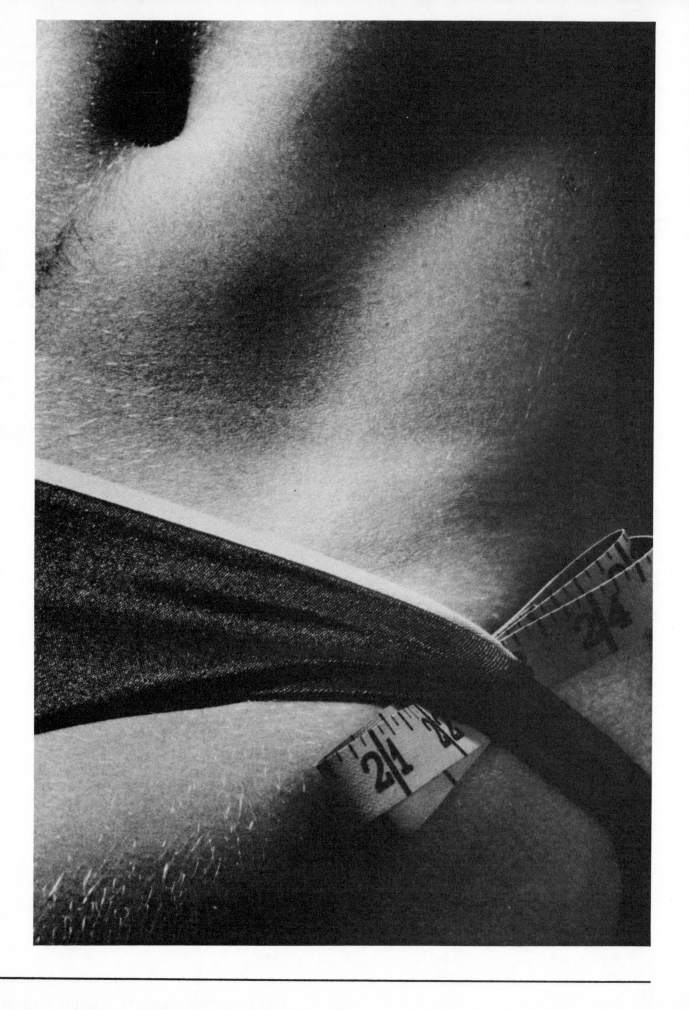

CHAPTER 2
FACTS ABOUT BODY FAT

"Starting tomorrow," the overweight woman announces, reaching for another piece of chocolate cake, "I'm going to lose this fat."

Do these words sound familiar? They should. Thousands of women decide to reduce every day. But even if these women do begin reducing tomorrow, their efforts will probably be in vain because they do not understand the fat they are fighting.

The Function of Body Fat

The primary function of body fat is the long-term storage of fuel. The use of fat for fuel did not originate with humans. Almost from the beginning of life on earth, fat has had a biological role to play as fuel storage for moving organisms. Larval forms of certain insects may carry 90 percent of their weight in lipid form. Locusts and monarch butterflies prepare for long-distance migrations by preflight feeding and fat depositing that can last several days. Before migrating, birds may fatten themselves by 25 percent in a week. Several species of fish, notably salmon and sharks, are recognized for their lipid reserves which provide energy for their long distance swims.

Human fat is distributed all over the body. But in spreading out under the skin, fat seems to take on new uses and begins to serve functions which may not have been intended in the evolutionary process. With a girdle of fat under the skin and around parts of the viscera, insulation and even heat production may be added to fat's primary use as a storage depot.

Types of Fat

There are three kinds of body fat: subcutaneous, depot, and essential.

Subcutaneous fat is the fat that lies in layers directly under the skin.

Depot fat is inherited fat deposited in certain areas of the body.

Essential fat is fat that cushions and protects many vital organs of the body.

About 50 percent of fat is subcutaneous, 40 percent is depot, and 10 percent is essential. A person can reduce subcutaneous and depot fat but not essential fat.

Unattractive Fat

In the last 40 years, it has become popular among physicians, insurance underwriters, psychotherapists, and fashion designers to attack obesity as a common enemy. Over the years, campaigns mustered in this cause have raised legions of specialists and specialties. A recent study done by an audience testing house confirmed the fact that 90 percent of the public does not like the way it looks. Americans, in fact, spend billions annually on diet and weight-reducing drugs, fat diet books, reducing machines, and health courses.

The bountiful supply of food in this country makes the ability of the body to store fat no longer a life-saving necessity. If anything, actuarial tables suggest that it may be just the opposite.

Insurance studies that ushered in a new world of body images for Americans were first published in 1912. As an indirect result, we are now taught that being over fat increases our chances of dying of heart disease, diabetes, and nephritis. Recently, asthma and homicide have been added to the list. There has been also the extra burden of psychological guilt produced by the fashion and sportsfitness industries. No one wants to take a fat girl out to dinner, do business with a butterball executive, or play racquetball with an obese partner.

The most recent figures published by the insurance companies suggest that almost 50 percent of the adult female population in the United States are seriously overweight. Figures for adult males run a close second. Experience has shown, however, that even if an average woman is at correct bodyweight for her height, it is very probable that she is still too fat for playing sports in the most efficient manner. And she is probably too fat for her potential physical beauty. Exercise physiology clinics that routinely measure and evaluate the body fat of women note that only once in a great while do they actually find a woman who is under fat. Over 99 percent of the women that they measure are too fat.

Evaluation of Body Fat

Seen under a microscope, fat tissue looks like a bubble bath. The globules are grouped together with stringy intercellular glue and streaked with a narrow filament of connective tissue, blood vessels, and nerves. This network of fat cells provides a living inner tube, inflatable or deflatable, with minimum stress to the skin and the viscera.

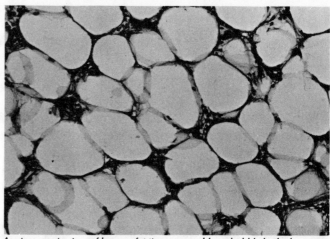

A microscopic view of human fat tissue resembles a bubble bath. A woman can increase the size and number of fat cells. But she can only decrease the size of the cells, never the number. It is much easier to prevent obesity than treat it.

Several methods have been used to measure body fat; x-rays, specific gravity, potassium 40, and skinfold thickness.

The easiest and most popular method is by measuring skinfold thickness. The thickness of a fold of skin in various areas of the body is measured with skinfold calipers. Such thickness data can be translated into percentage of body fat. Although these data are not perfect or totally precise they do give a better indication of the amount of body fat than mere bodyweight and height comparisons.

The amount of body fat varies with age and sex. It is greatest in infancy, diminshes in childhood, and increases again during adolescence. Research indicates that girls and women normally have more body fat than do boys and men. An abnormally great or small amount of body fat is related to good or poor nutritional status, especially when compared with bodyweight.

An individual can obtain a fair estimate of her body fat by the "pinch test". The following procedure applies to both men and women:

Directions
1. Have a friend do the pinching and measuring. A woman cannot measure her own skinfold.
2. Let the right arm hang down to the side.
3. Locate the skinfold site on the back of the upper arm midway between the shoulder and the elbow.
4. Grasp a vertical fold of skin between the thumb

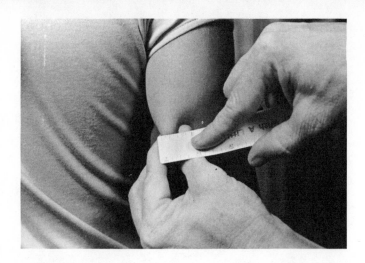

and first finger. Pull the skin and fat away from the arm.

Make sure the fold does not include any muscle, just skin and fat. Practice pinching and pulling the skin until there is no muscle included.

Most Americans have over 25 percent of their bodyweight in fat. Athletes have a smaller percentage of fat than non-athletes. An ideal amount of body fat for most men is below 12 percent. The average female interested in a slender figure should strive for below 18 percent body fat.

Inherited Patterns of Fat Distribution

Just as different families have characteristic patterns of fat distribution, so do different races. Perhaps the best known racial variant of fat patterns is that of the African Hottentot and Bushman. If the women become obese, the bulk of their fat is deposited as a great mound around the buttocks. The mound may actually grow to the size of a large watermelon while the woman remains relatively lean over the rest of her body.

Percent of Fat -- Men		
Skinfold Thickness (inches)		Percentage
¼	=	5-9
½	=	9-13
¾	=	13-18
1	=	18-22
1¼	=	22-27

Percent of Fat -- Women		
Skinfold Thickness (inches)		Percentage
¼	=	8-13
½	=	13-18
¾	=	18-23
1	=	23-28
1¼	=	28-33

5. Measure with a ruler the thickness of the skinfold to the nearest ¼ inch.

Be sure to measure the distance between the thumb and the finger. Sometimes the top of the skinfold is thicker than the distance between the thumb and the finger. To avoid this make sure the top of the skinfold is level with the top of the thumb. Do not press the ruler against the skinfold. This will flatten it out and make it appear thicker than it really is.

6. Take two separate measures of skinfold thickness, releasing the skin between each measure, to determine the average thickness.

Skinfold #1 _____ Skinfold #2 _____

Average skinfold _____.

7. Calculate the average skinfold thickness and use the above chart to estimate percentage of body fat.

Hormones also influence the distribution of body fat. Androgens and estrogens are largely responsible for the difference in the way men and women deposit fat. The breasts are mostly fat, not glandular tissue as many people imagine, and estrogens are particularly responsible for this fat distribution.

Men, as they grow older, tend to deposit their fat more frontally than do women. Women tend to deposit their fat more on the back of the body. This is true not only for that percentage of fat that accumulates in their buttocks, but also for the lower part of their backs.

Another genetic difference in fat distribution between men and women is that men tend to deposit more of their fat on the trunk rather than

BASICS: FACTS ABOUT BODY FAT

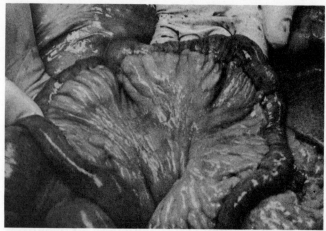
An over-fat person not only stores fat directly under the skin, but also around the internal organs. This photograph, which was taken during and autopsy, revels a large amount of fat around the intestines.

on the arms and legs as women do. Male fat is usually truncal fat as well as frontal.

Much of the adipose tissue that a man accumulates on his front will be concentrated above the navel in that low-slung beer belly. Fat women usually concentrate their truncal fat below the navel and over the hips.

Losing Fat Slowly

It is virtually impossible to lose body fat quickly and easily. Almost anyone can lose five or ten pounds of bodyweight on a short-term basis. But unless the process is slow, most of the weight loss will be from the muscles and organs rather than from fat stores. What counts is losing weight permanently and making sure that the weight loss is fat. This requires discipline, motivation, and patience.

Advertising Offering Fast Weight Loss

A large percentage of advertising in popular magazines offering fast weight loss is myth, half truths, and outright lies. Many of them advocate dangerous practices. Some of the more popular ones peddling miraculous ways to lose fat are as follows:

• A weighted belt an individual can wear to "Whittle inches off his waist." This is a useless gadget according to the Federal Trade Commission which also says that by wearing the weighted belt some individuals "could physically injure themselves."

• An electrical device that transmits current to the muscles through contact pads strapped to the body. Actually the muscle movements are too small to consume enough energy to cause a noticeable reduction in fat. Doctors believe these machines can be dangerous to the heart and other organs that can respond to electrical stimuli.

• A mechanical vibrating belt may relax a woman and make her feel better, but it certainly will not remove fat. Fat cannot be shaken, tickled, beaten, or stroked from the body.

• Rubber clothes, which range from belts, shorts, and shirts to full outfits, that are supposed to sweat off the fat and inches. Any weight loss from it is simply a result of dehydration, which is quickly replaced when the woman quenches her thirst. Since fat contains just a small percent of water, none of the loss comes from the person's body fat.

• Sauna wraps for particular parts of the body. In this idea, the specific part a woman wants reduced is wrapped with tape, which has been soaked in a "secret" solution. The woman sits in a sauna bath for 30 minutes, and supposedly the secret solution draws the excess fat from the body. Again, fat cannot be removed from the body by sweating.

• Cellulite remedies for removing fat around a woman's hips and thighs. Cellulite is a trade word supposedly connoting a unique type of fat that can only be removed by costly and elaborate procedures. But cellulite is not a special type of fat. It is just plain fat. The relationship between the skin, the fat, and the underlying muscles and fasciae are distinctive in human beings. Other species have fur, feathers, and certain vascular blood-shunting devices to combat cold weather. But we humans have virtually nothing between us and the elements except fat and skin. This may be one of the reasons that fat adheres so stubbornly to our underlying fasciae.

It is this adhesiveness that accounts for the kind of dimpling effect that has been dubbed "cellulite." The term has been applied to the puckering or dimpling of fat that occurs in the buttocks and thighs of over fat and usually middle aged women. Although there is no such word medically, "cellulite" has become such a common term that it would be pointless to try to remove it from the dieter's vocabulary.

In cellulite, the connective tissue which serves as pouches for large groups of fat cells in a honeycomb arrangement under the skin lose their elasticity and shrink with age. The overlying skin which is attached to these fibers then contracts. If the size of the fat cells encased in them does not shrink to match, a kind of overall dimpling appears on the surface of the skin.

The cure for this is to reduce the size of the pouched fat by dieting. A fat woman's goal should be to shrink the fat cells inside the pockets of connective tissue down to the limits of the shrunken connective tissue.

The American Medical Association has issued a statement calling cellulite a hoax and denounces its remedies as economic exploitation.

• Over-the-counter drugs that claim to cause quick fat loss. Despite the efforts of the pharmaceutical industry, no satisfactory fat-reducing drug has been developed. Nobody will lose fat simply by consuming a certain capsule, tablet, or pill. In the opinion of many physicians the over-the-counter weight-losing and appetite control claims are nonsense and lies. They should be withdrawn from the market.

Consumer Protection

Newspapers and magazines have the First Amendment right of freedom of speech. But this freedom combined with commercially motivated advertising concerning quick and easy ways to lose fat result in the deception of many consumers. The clever promoter knows that he can advertise almost anything with impunity in any conceivable way for a surprisingly long time.

The woman must realize that no one is going to protect her from untrue advertisements and their products. She must rely on her own judgement to guard against fitness fraud. Scientific facts clearly show that there is no quick and easy way to lose body fat.

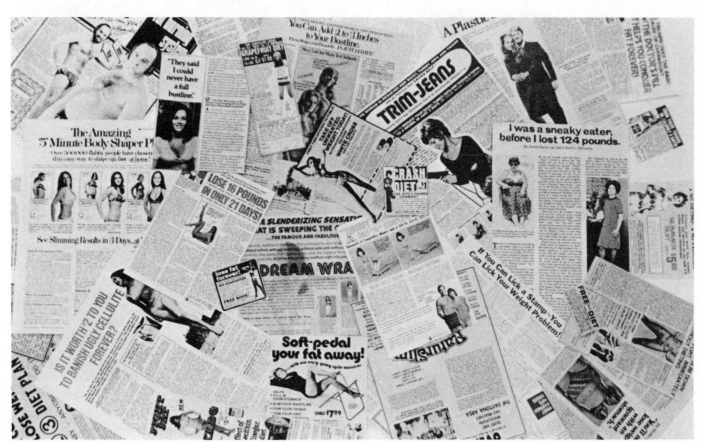

Despite the promises in these advertisements, there is no quick and easy way to lose fat.

23

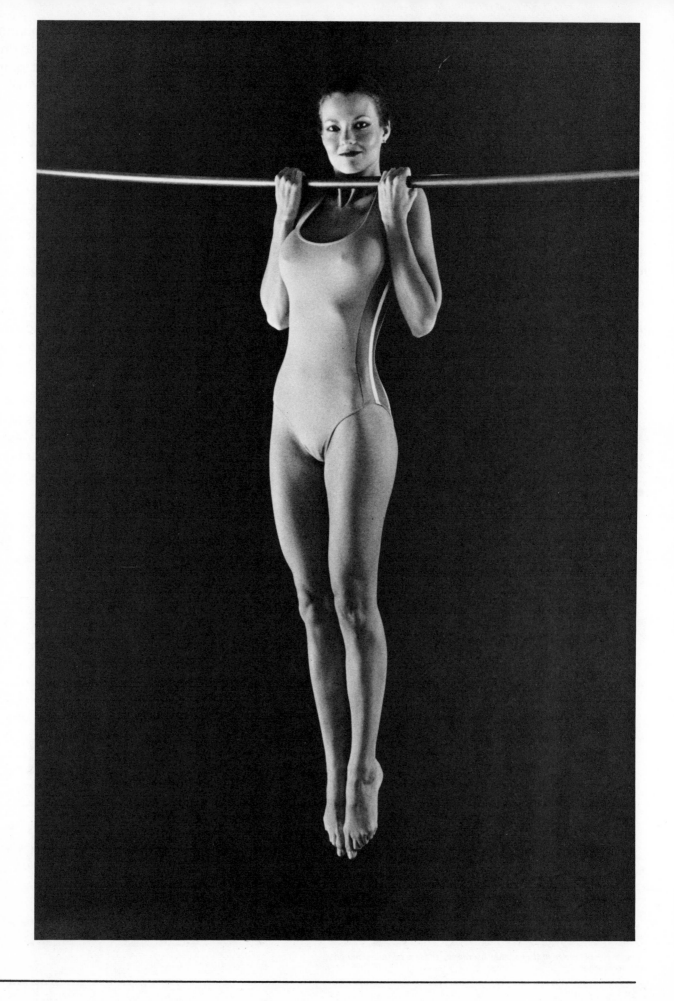

CHAPTER 3
BODY-SHAPING FUNDA-MENTALS

"**Y**ou must first learn the fundamentals." This is the challenge every instructor flings at any student who comes in.

Proficiency in shaping and strengthening the feminine body is the same as in mathematics, tennis, cooking, and every other subject. The student must begin with the fundamentals. A clear understanding of the following fundamentals will assure the best possible results from the exercises described in this book.

Exercise Equipment

There is nothing a woman has to buy for the basic body-shaping program. The equipment is easily available around her house. The following items will be needed:
2 kitchen chairs with flat backs
1 strong broom handle
1 small bench
2 medium-sized cans of vegetables. These should weigh about two pounds each.
2 plastic bottles with sculptured handles. The one-gallon size full of water weighs about 9 pounds. The weight can be lowered by using less water.
1 medium-sized bath towel

The two chairs can be used as parallel bars to support the body's weight in various exercise. The broomstick laid across the backs of the chairs can be a horizontal bar to support the weight of the body or to simulate a barbell. Lying across a bench often provides a more effective means of exercise than lying on the floor. The plastic bottles and cans of vegetables make excellent weights to hold in the hands. A few partner exercises can be performed with a towel.

After several months of exercising with homemade equipment , a woman may want to purchase a small adjustable barbell and dumbbell set. This will increase the effectiveness of the routine, and it will allow for greater variation in exercise.

An alternative to buying weights is to join a fitness club. The serious woman should be sure that the people in the club know the value of heavy

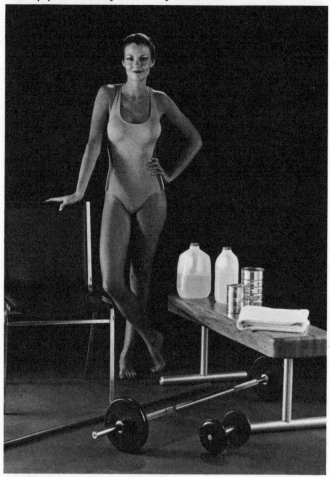

exercise for women. Passive machines and low-intensity exercise produce poor results. The well-equipped fitness club will encourage women to train with barbells and dumbbells, or Nautilus machines.

Intensity

The improvement of body shape is proportionate to the intensity of exercise. The higher the intensity, the more the muscles are stimulated. Performing an exercise to the point of momentary muscular failure assures that the individual has trained to maximum intensity. Muscular failure means that no additional repetitions of the exercise are possible. It is only by working to this extent that the woman engages a maximum number of muscle fibers.

The first few repetitions are merely preparation, doing little to increase strength. These repetitions are of limited value because the intensity is low. The final repetitions are productive because the intensity is high.

Many women refuse to perform these last several repetitions. But those forced repetitions are the most effective. An exercise should not be considered completed until the individual cannot perform another repetition in correct form.

Progression

The cornerstone of body shaping is progression. Progression means attempting to increase the work load every training session. With each workout, the individual should try to add another repetition, additional resistance, or both. Experience has shown that at least 8 repetitions should be performed, but not more than 12. If she cannot achieve 8 repetitions, the resistance is too heavy. If she can perform more than 12 repetitions, it is too light. When the trainee can perform 12 repetitions or more, it is the signal to increase the resistance on that exercise by approximately 5 percent at the next workout.

Form

Repetitions performed in a slow, smooth manner apply steady force through the entire movement. Fast repetitions apply force to only a small portion at the beginning and the end of the movement. When a resistance is jerked or thrown three or four times, the actual force is directed to the joints and muscles. This is both ineffective and dangerous.

The range of movement of each repetition, from full extension to full flexion, should be as great as possible. To contract at all, a muscle must produce movement. To contract fully, it must produce a full range of movement. If the movement resulting from muscular contraction is less than full range, the entire length of the muscle is not involved in the work. Improved body shape is most likely when the muscles have been strengthened in every position over a full range of possible movement.

Accentuate the Negative

For best results, each repetition should be performed in a negative-emphasized manner. The performance of weight training requires the raising and lowering of resistance. When a woman raises a weight, she moves against the resistance of gravity and performs positive work.

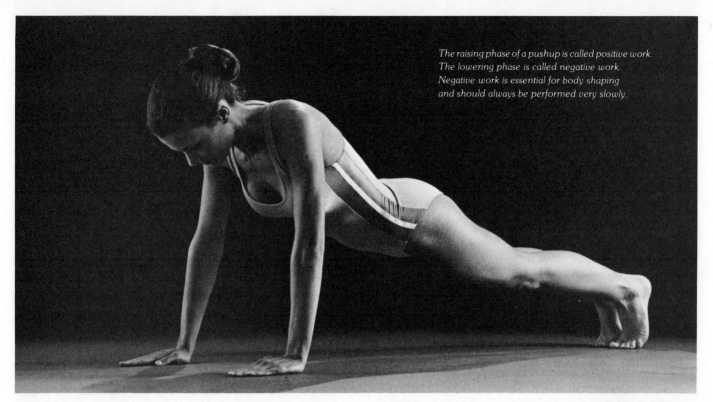

Lowering a weight under control brings gravity into play in another fashion. The lowering portion of an exercise is termed negative work.

In a pushup she performs both positive and negative work during each repetition. Positive resistance straightens the arms and raises her body. Negative resistance bends the arms and lowers her body. Up is positive, down is negative. This is true in all forms of exercise.

Physiological research has recently determined that for body-shaping and strength-building purposes, the negative part of an exercise has much more value than the positive portion. Exercises, therefore, should accentuate the negative part of every movement.

In normal exercise, a woman should always concentrate on the lowering part of the movement. If it takes two seconds to lift a weight smoothly, it should take about four seconds to lower it.

To perform negative-only exercise, the woman needs to select a heavier weight than she can lift. Initially she should use about 40 percent more weight than she can handle for 10 repetitions in a normal manner. With this additional amount of weight, she has one or two assistants lift the barbell. It is then her job to lower the resistance back to the starting position.

During the first two or three repetitions, it should take approximately 8 to 10 seconds per repetition to lower the resistance in a slow, even manner. It should be possible for the trainee to stop and reverse the movement of these repetitions although no attempt should be made to do so.

If the weight has been correctly selected, the middle three or four repetitions should be performed slightly faster, approximately 4 or 5 seconds per repetition. In these repetitions, the individual should be able to stop the movement.

During the last repetitions, it becomes impossible to stop the downward movement. The exercise is finally terminated when the downward movement can no longer be controlled.

Properly performed, negative-only exercise is a very effective style of training. But most women need someone to lift the barbell for them.

A few exercises can be performed in a negative-only manner with help. Negative chins and dips can be done by climbing into the top position with

BASICS: BODY-SHAPING FUNDAMENTALS

the legs and slowly lowering with the arms. Thus, the lower body is doing the positive work and the upper body is doing the negative work. Pushups, situps, and a few other freehand exercises can be performed in this fashion also.

Duration

If each exercise is done properly in a high-intensity fashion, brief workouts must be the rule. High-intensity exercise has an effect on the entire system that can be either beneficial or damaging. Low-intensity work has practically no effect. Body shaping is improved by high-intensity work followed by an adequate period of rest. Intensive work, however, must not be overdone.

Many women mistakenly perform too much exercise. They do too many different movements, too many sets, and too many workouts within a given period of time. When an excess of exercise is performed, total recovery between workouts becomes impossible. So does high-intensity training.

A woman can perform brief and infrequent high-intensity exercise or long and frequent low-intensity workouts. But she cannot perform long and frequent exercise at a high level of intensity. That will bring unsatisfactory results. It can also lead to total exhaustion.

Understanding the requirements for a productive style of high-intensity exercise allows selection of the best exercises for a particular purpose. In most cases, not more than 12 different exercises should be performed in any one workout. The lower body should have 4-6 exercises and the upper body 6-8.

A set of 10 repetitions performed in proper style should take about one minute to complete. Allowing one minute between exercises, most women should be able to complete 12 exercises in less than 25 minutes. As she works into better condition, the time between exercises should be reduced. It is entirely possible to go through an entire workout of 12 exercises in less than 15 minutes. Such a workout not only develops muscular shape and strength, but also a high level of heart-lung endurance.

More is Not Better

A physically fit woman does not need more exercise than a beginner. Rather, the need changes to more strenuous but less exercise.

Beginners usually show acceptable strength gains on most types of exercise programs, even though they may perform several sets of more than 12 repetitions in each training session. They are able to make this progress, at least for a while, because they are not strong enough to use up all their recovery ability. As they get stronger, however, they do use that recovery ability, and their progress stops. The stronger the woman becomes, the greater resistance she handles and the greater inroads she makes into her recovery ability. So the advanced trainee must reduce her overall exercise from 12 to 10, and train only at high intensity twice a week. On Monday, she might train to exhaustion, on Wednesday less strenuously, and on Friday, strenuously again.

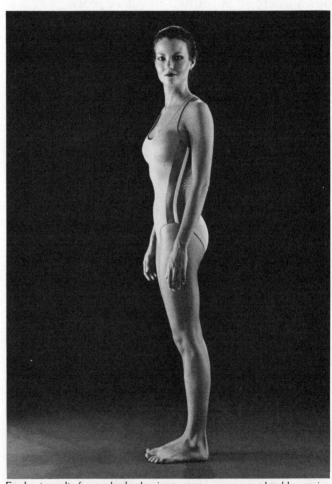

For best results from a body-shaping program, a woman should exercise her larger muscles first and her smaller muscles last.

The Wednesday workout will not stimulate strength increases, but it will keep her muscles from atrophying. It will permit improvement by not making significant inroads into the woman's recovery ability.

Order

Workouts should begin with the largest muscle groups and proceed downward to the smallest. This is important for two reasons. One, working the largest muscles first brings the greatest degree of overall body stimulation. Two, it is impossible to reach momentary muscular exhaustion in a large muscle if the smaller muscle group serving as a link between the resistance and the larger muscle groups has been previously exhausted. Thus, it is important to work the largest muscles while the system is still capable of working with the desired intensity.

For best results, the order of exercise should be as follows:
1. Hips and buttocks
2. Legs
3. Torso
4. Arms
5. Waist
6. Neck and face

Frequency

A woman should rest at least 48 hours, but not more than 96 hours between body-shaping workouts.

High-intensity exercise causes a complex chemical reaction inside a muscle. If given time, the muscle will compensate by strengthening certain cells. High-intensity exercise, therefore, is necessary to stimulate figure shaping. But that is not the only requisite. The stimulated muscle must be given time to improve.

Research has shown that there should be approximately 48 hours between workouts, but 72 to 96 hours between sessions are required for extremely strong athletes. High levels of muscular size and strength begin to decrease and atrophy after 96 hours of normal activity. This means that a woman should exercise every other day.

An every-other-day, three-times-per-week program also seems to provide the body with the needed irregularity of training. A first workout is performed on Monday. Two days later, the second workout comes on Wednesday, and the third on Friday. Thus, on Sunday, the system is excited and is prepared for a fourth workout, but it does not come. Instead, it is a day later, on the next Monday when the body is neither expecting nor prepared for it. This schedule of training prevents the body from falling into a regular routine. Since the system is never quite able to adjust to this irregularity of training, improvement is stimulated.

Keeping Accurate Records

The serious trainee should keep accurate records of her workout-by-workout progress. This can be done on a card that lists the exercises with ample space to the right for recording the date, resistance, repetitions, and training time.

Rating the Exercise

Potential benefits of exercise are largely determined by two factors: the quantity of movement by a specific part of the body and the quality of the resistance applied against it. The exercises in the next eight chapters are given a rating of A, B, or C according to these two factors.
A -- An "A" rating signifies that an exercise provides effective resistance and a great range of movement for a particular part of the body.
B -- A "B" rating means that the exercise provides either effective resistance of a great range or movement, but not both.
C -- A "C" rating indicates that the exercise is of limited benefit. These exercises are included because they are better than no exercise at all. They should be used only in lieu of working with the required equipment or when conditions prevent the performance of A or B-rated exercises.

In chapters 4-11, the exercises listed and described with photographic illustrations overlap to some extent. A certain exercise may benefit more than one part of the body and thus be included in more than one chapter.

Warming Up

Warming up is a safeguard against injury. On the warm-up, the cartilages of the knee increase their thickness and provide a better fit for the surface of the knee joint. Friction-like resistance of the muscle cells is reduced by the higher temperature of the body. The elasticity of the tendons and ligaments is also increased. It is this change to higher temperature that augments speed of movement, expands power potential, and minimizes risk of injury.

A few degrees' rise in temperature of the muscle cells accelerates the production of energy by one-third. These changes in the human mechanism are similar to those that occur in an automobile as it warms up.

Almost any sequence of light calisthenic movements can be used as a general warm-up to precede a vigorous body-shaping session.

Words of Caution

Before beginning a body-shaping program, a woman should have a medical examination. Vigorous exercise can be dangerous to some people. Intense physical activity coupled with certain environmental conditions may aggravate existing asthmatic conditions. People with a tendency toward high blood pressure should be closely supervised in any heavy lifting or straining exercises that may cause temporary increases in that pressure. Those over the age of 35, and coronary-prone younger people who possess high-risk factors, should obtain a stress-test electrocardiogram. Stress tests are particularly important to those who have the following risk factors: overweight, hypertension, diabetes, sedentary lifestyle, cigarette smoking, and a family history of early heart disease.

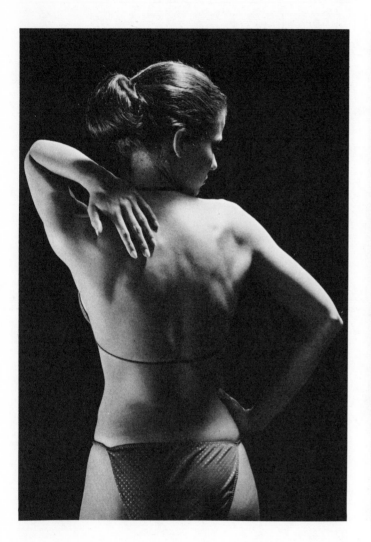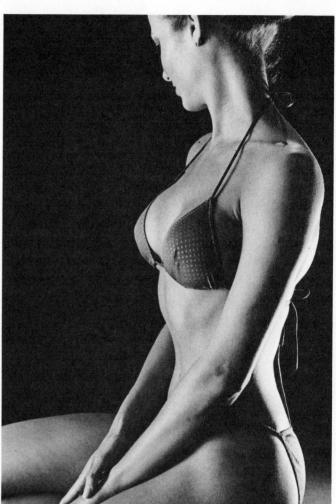

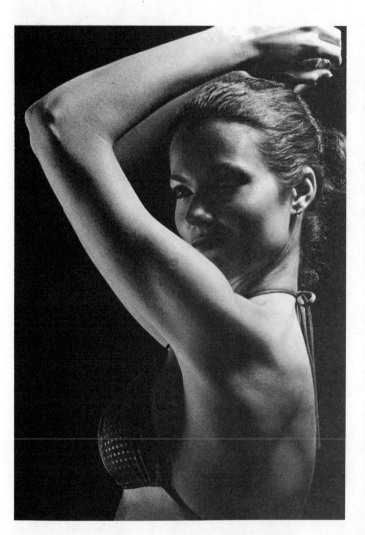
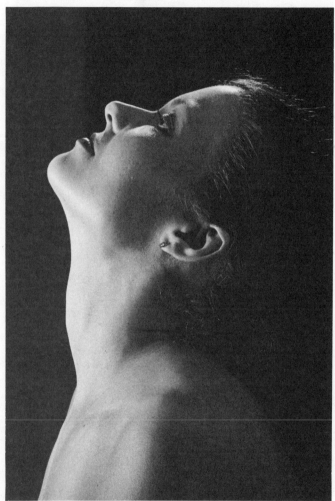

II. BODY SHAPING

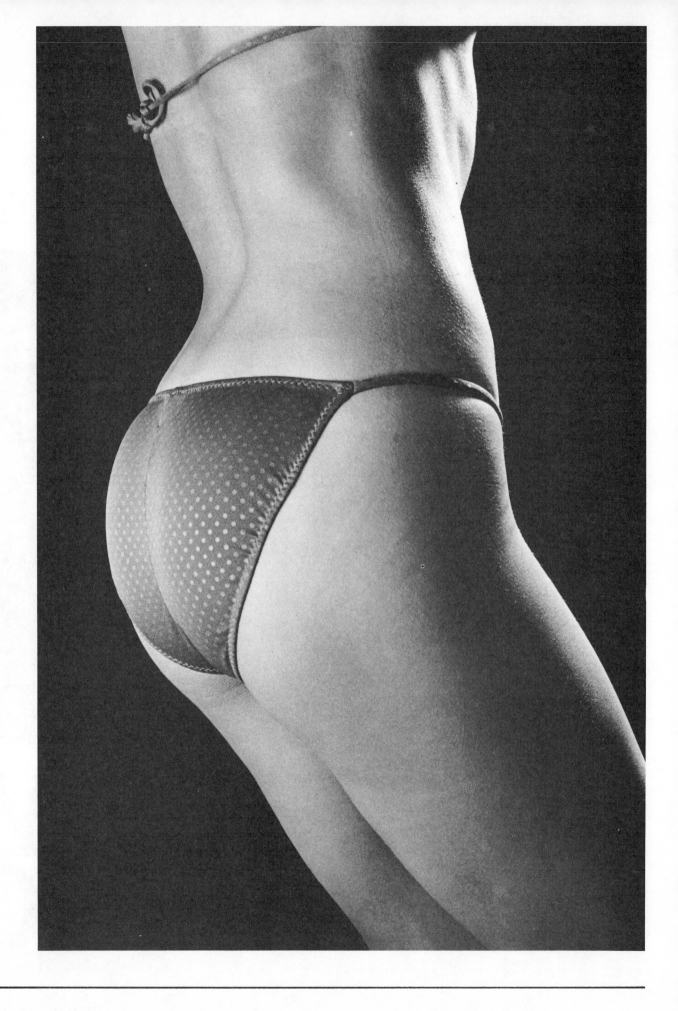

CHAPTER 4
HIPS & BUTTOCKS

Dimples, pock marks and ripples on the buttocks and hips may be the first sign that the body is getting out of shape. What started out as pleasing curves on a woman's body may now be a sagging mass of tissue and fat. The average woman can diet until she starves, but it will be all in vain.

Those dimple formations and sagging behinds are not the result of improper diet. They are the result of shrinking muscles and connective tissue. Most women spend too much time sitting and not enough in vigorous exercise. Proper exercise is the answer to a more shapely and firmer posterior. The real secret, however, is the kind and quantity of exercise. Specific exercises to condition the hips require an understanding of the anatomical composition of the buttocks.

Anatomy of the Buttocks

Starting in the middle of the hips and working toward the back, a large bone formation constitutes the pelvic girdle. Connected to the pelvic girdle are 22 major and minor muscles. The most important muscle of this group from the standpoint of buttock strength, shape, and size is the gluteal group, of which the gluteus maximus is the largest. The major function of this muscle is the extension of the hip, but only under certain conditions. In easy walking, the muscle remains relaxed and will remain so until the individual tries to walk very fast, jump, walk upstairs, run or push something. The general rule seems to be that the gluteus maximus is not called into action in the movement of the upper leg until the hip is flexed in excess of 45 degrees.

Few people are involved in a consistent program of intense exercise after they have finished high school. As a result, the dimples and flabby muscles are just around the corner. Women suffer more than men from this condition because their hip widths are greater, and they generally have a higher percentage of body fat than men.

From an athletic point of view, the buttocks are the largest and strongest muscle of the entire body. They are by far the most important muscles for running and jumping. From 65 to 80 percent of the power to run and jump comes from the intense contractions of these muscles.

Whether a women is concerned about buttocks shape and strength from a cosmetic or athletic viewpoint, experience proves that these large muscles respond very quickly to proper exercise.

BODY SHAPING

EXERCISE:
SQUAT WITH PLASTIC BOTTLES

RATING: A
EQUIPMENT:
WATER-FILLED PLASTIC BOTTLES

Starting Position: Stand erect, feet shoulder-width apart, with a bottle in each hand. The feet should be flat if working the back is desired. The heels should be elevated if working the calves is preferable.

Movement: Slowly lower the upper body by bending the knees and hips. Look straight ahead or slightly upward during the movement. Continue downward until the thighs come into contact with the backs of the calves. **Do not** relax or bounce at the bottom of the movement. Return smoothly to the starting position and repeat.

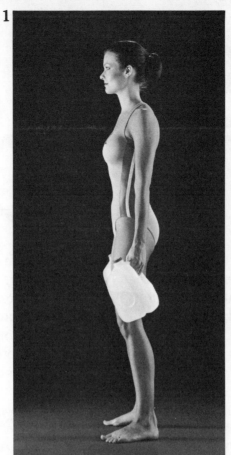
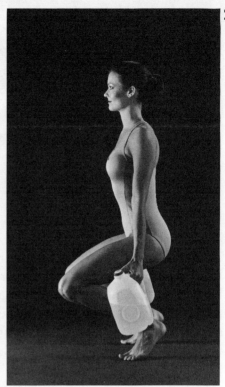

EXERCISE:
ONE-LEGGED SQUAT

RATING: A
EQUIPMENT:
CHAIR

Starting Position: Grasp the back of a straight chair with the right hand and hold the right leg in front of the body. Do not let the right foot touch the floor. Stand erect. Keep the foot flat if working the back is desired. Keep the heel elevated if working the calf is preferable.

Movement: Slowly lower the upper body by bending the left knee and hip. Look straight ahead or slightly upward during the movement. Continue downward until the back of the left thigh comes into contact with the left calf. **Do not** bounce at the bottom of the movement. **Do not** relax at the bottom of the movement. Return smoothly to the starting position and repeat. Work the right leg in the same manner.

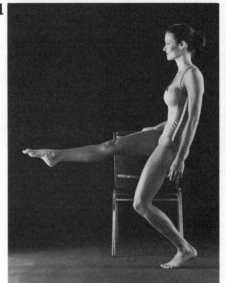
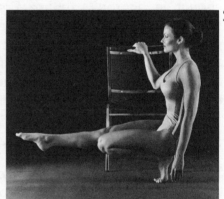

EXERCISE:
NEGATIVE-EMPHASIZED SQUAT WITH PARTNER

RATING: A
EQUIPMENT: PARTNER

Starting Position: Stand erect with the feet shoulder-width apart. From behind, a partner places his hands on the squatter's shoulders.

Movement: As the knees bend the partner applies pressure downward. Very slow movements are called for in this exercise. At the bottom position, the pressure is removed and the squatter returns to the top position where the partner resumes the negative resistance.

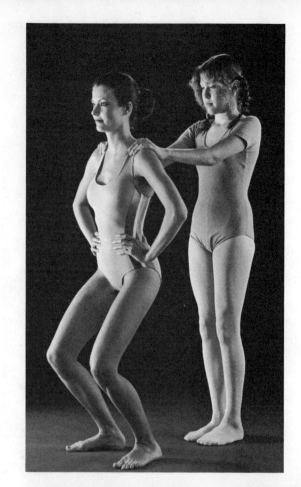

EXERCISE:
BARBELL SQUAT

RATING: A
EQUIPMENT: BARBELL

Starting Position: Stand erect, feet shoulder-width apart, with a barbell securely in the hands and balanced across the shoulders. The feet should be flat if working the back is desired. The heels should be elevated if working the calves is preferable.

Movement: Slowly lower the upper body by bending the knees and hips. Look straight ahead or slightly upward during the movement. Continue downward until the thighs come into contact with the backs of the calves. **Do not** relax or bounce at the bottom of the movement. Return smoothly to the starting position and repeat.

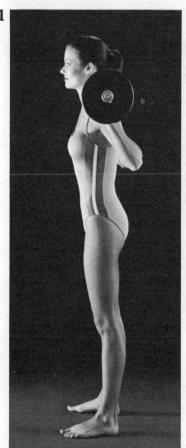

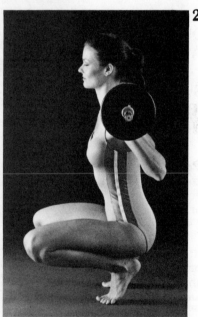

EXERCISE:
CHAIR STEP-UP
WITH PLASTIC
BOTTLE

RATING: A
EQUIPMENT:
ONE CHAIR AND ONE
WATER-FILLED
PLASTIC BOTTLE

Starting Position: Stand erect with the left foot planted firmly in a straight-bottomed chair and the other on the floor. The bottle is held in one hand.

Movement: Slowly step up onto the chair, then step down with the same leg and up again until it is completely fatigued. Switch sides and step up with the other leg.

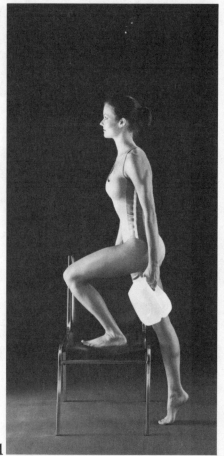
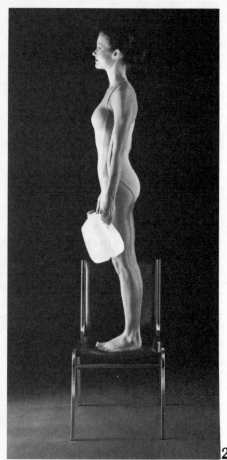

EXERCISE:
HIP ADDUCTION
WITH PARTNER

RATING: A
EQUIPMENT:
PARTNER

Starting Position: Sit on the floor facing a partner. Both should lean back, using the elbows for support. Keep the legs straight. Place the ankles outside the partner's ankles.

Movement: Squeeze the legs forcibly together against the partner's attempt to spread them. The partner provides both positive and negative resistance, which is felt in the groin and inner thigh area. Repeat.

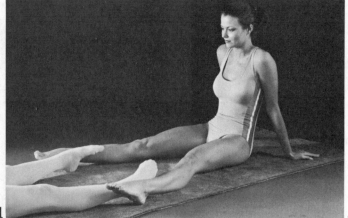
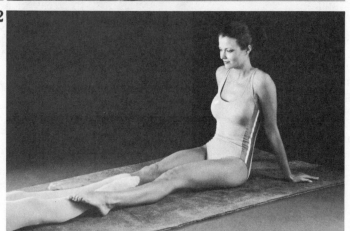

EXERCISE:
HIP ABDUCTION WITH PARTNER

RATING: A

EQUIPMENT: PARTNER

Starting Position: Sit on the floor facing a partner. Both should lean back, using the elbows for support. Keep the legs straight. Place the ankles inside the partner's ankles.

Movement: Spread the legs forcibly against the partner's squeezing resistance. The partner should allow positive and negative work of this spreading function. This is felt in the outer hips. Repeat until fatigued.

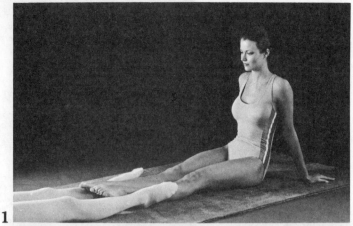

1

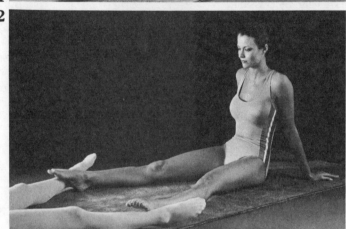

2

EXERCISE:
SQUAT

RATING: B

EQUIPMENT: NONE

Starting Position: Stand erect with the heels flat. The feet should be shoulder-width apart.

Movement: Lower the body by bending the knees as far as possible. Keep the back vertical. Return to the starting position and repeat. **Do not** bounce or relax at the bottom of the movement.

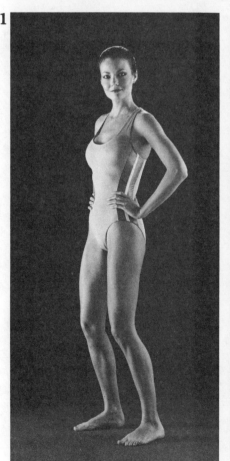

1

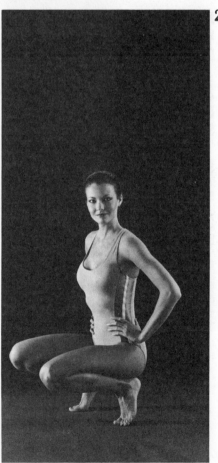

2

BODY SHAPING: HIPS AND BUTTOCKS

EXERCISE:
WIDE SQUAT

RATING: B

EQUIPMENT:
NONE

Starting Position: Place the feet twice shoulder-width apart and turn the toes outward. Stand erect with the heels flat. Rest the hands on the head.

Movement: Lower the body by bending the knees as far as possible. Keep the back vertical. Return to starting position and repeat. **Do not** bounce or relax at the bottom of the movement.

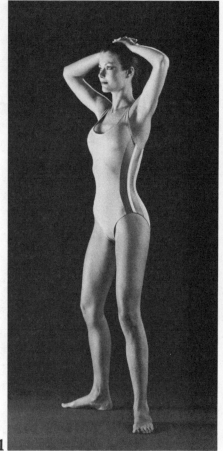
1

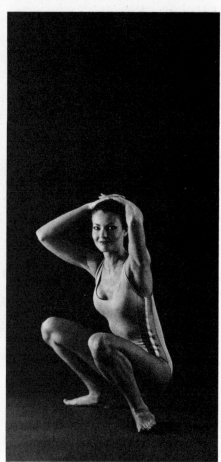
2

EXERCISE:
WALL LEG
PRESS

RATING: B

EQUIPMENT:
SMOOTH WALL

Starting Position: Stand erect and lean back against a smooth, sturdy wall. Both heels should be approximately one-foot away from the wall, and shoulder-width apart. A cushion may be placed at the bottom of the wall.

Movement: Bend at the knees and slide the body down the wall. The object of the wall leg press is to descend as slowly as possible for one repetition. The movement gets more difficult as the body lowers. An adequate lowering time is from 30 to 60 seconds.

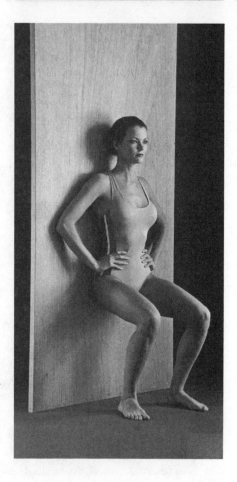

EXERCISE:
LUNGE WITH PLASTIC BOTTLES

RATING: B
EQUIPMENT:
WATER-FILLED PLASTIC BOTTLES

Starting Position: With plastic bottles at arms length to the sides, stand erect. Place the left foot in front of the right. The wider the feet are placed, the more stretch in the exercise.

Movement: Keeping the right leg straight, lower the body by bending the left leg at the knee. **Do not** relax at the bottom of the movement or bounce. The back should remain vertical as it moves forward. Straighten the left leg and repeat. When completed, switch to right leg.

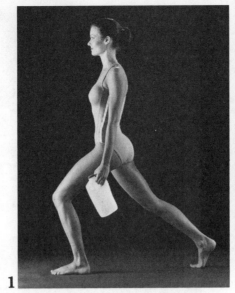
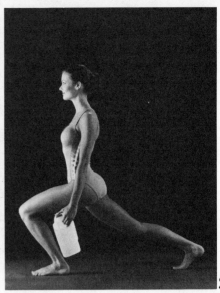

EXERCISE:
CHAIR STEP-UP

RATING: B
EQUIPMENT:
CHAIR

Starting Position: Stand erect with the foot planted firmly in a straight-bottom chair and the other on the floor.

Movement: Slowly step up onto the chair, then step down with the left leg until it is completely fatigued. Switch sides and step up with the right leg.

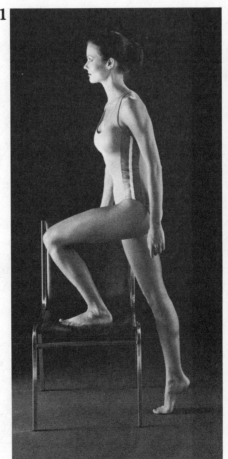
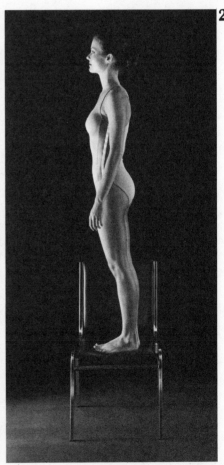

BODY SHAPING: HIPS AND BUTTOCKS

EXERCISE:
REVERSE LEG RAISE

RATING: B
EQUIPMENT: NONE

Starting Position: Lie face-down on the floor. The hands should be by the hips.

Movement: Lift both legs backward as high as possible. Pause briefly at the highest position and strongly squeeze the buttocks together. Slowly return the legs to the floor and repeat.

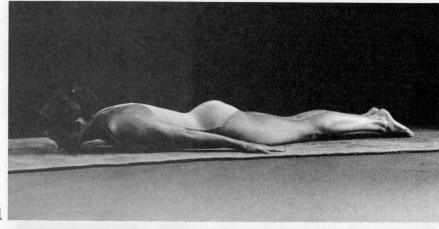

1

2

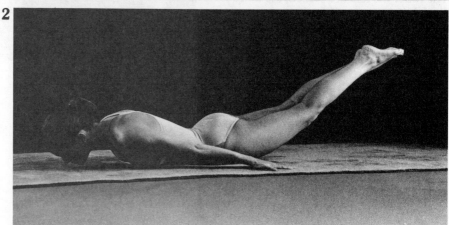

EXERCISE:
HIP EXTENSION

RATING: B
EQUIPMENT: NONE

Starting position: Assume a crawling stance on the hands and knees.

Movement: Slowly pull the left knee to the chest, then extend it high above and behind the back. Straighten the leg at the end of the movement. Pause and lower slowly to the chest and repeat. The right leg should be worked after the left is fatigued.

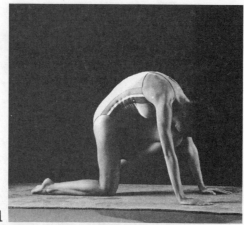

1

2

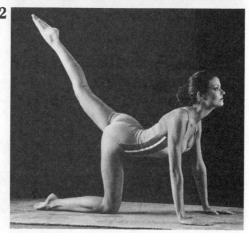

EXERCISE:
BENT-KNEED SITUP

RATING: B
EQUIPMENT:
PARTNER

Starting Position: Sit on the floor with the knees together and bent. Instruct a partner to hold the feet in place. Interlace the hands behind the head. Movement is easier with arms across the chest.

Movement: Slowly raise the torso from the floor until the chest touches the knees. Return to the starting position and repeat.

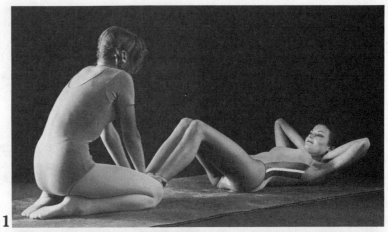

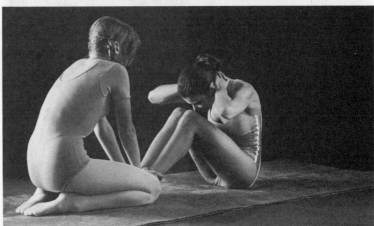

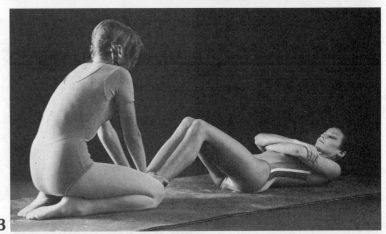

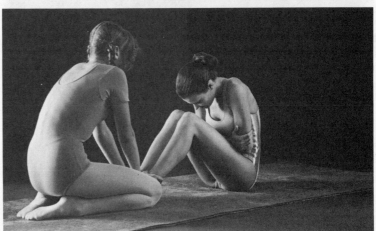

43

BODY SHAPING: HIPS AND BUTTOCKS

EXERCISE:
STATIC CHAIR SQUEEZE

RATING: C
EQUIPMENT: CHAIR

Starting Position: Lie on the floor with the legs up, knees bent, in front of the torso. Place a chair between the knees so that the chair's legs contact the inner thighs just above the knees.

Movement: Attempt to squeeze the knees together against the chair legs. Hold for a count of three and release. Perform 8-12 times.

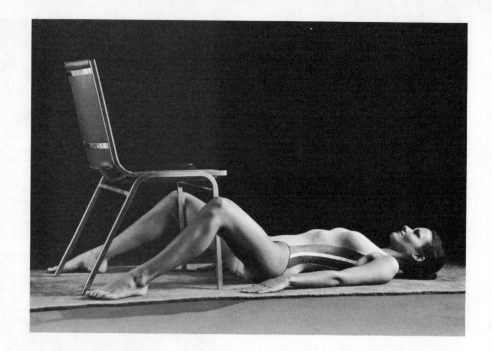

EXERCISE:
STATIC CHAIR SPREAD

RATING: C
EQUIPMENT: CHAIR

Starting Position: Lie on the floor with the legs up, knees bent, in front of the torso and between the legs of a chair. The feet should be on the floor and the chair legs should contact slightly above the outer knees.

Movement: Attempt to spread the knees against the chair legs. Hold for a count of three, release and repeat 8-12 times.

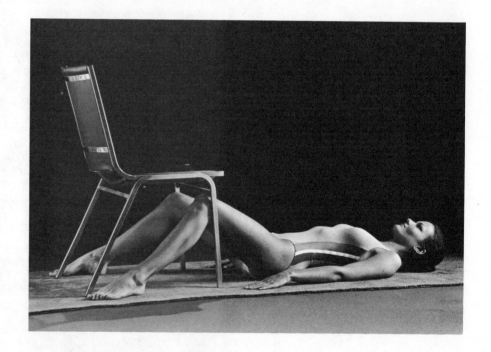

EXERCISE:
STANDING THIGH RAISE

RATING: C
EQUIPMENT: NONE

Starting Position: Stand on the left leg.

Movement: Raise and lower the right thigh against resistance provided by right hand. Try to achieve the highest possible position with the thigh. Perform 8-12 repetitions with the right, then, 8-12 with the left.

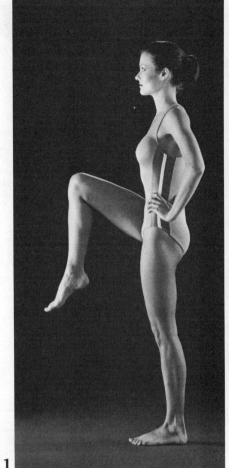

1

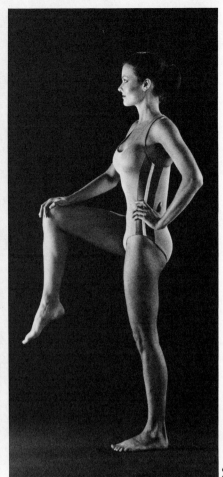

2

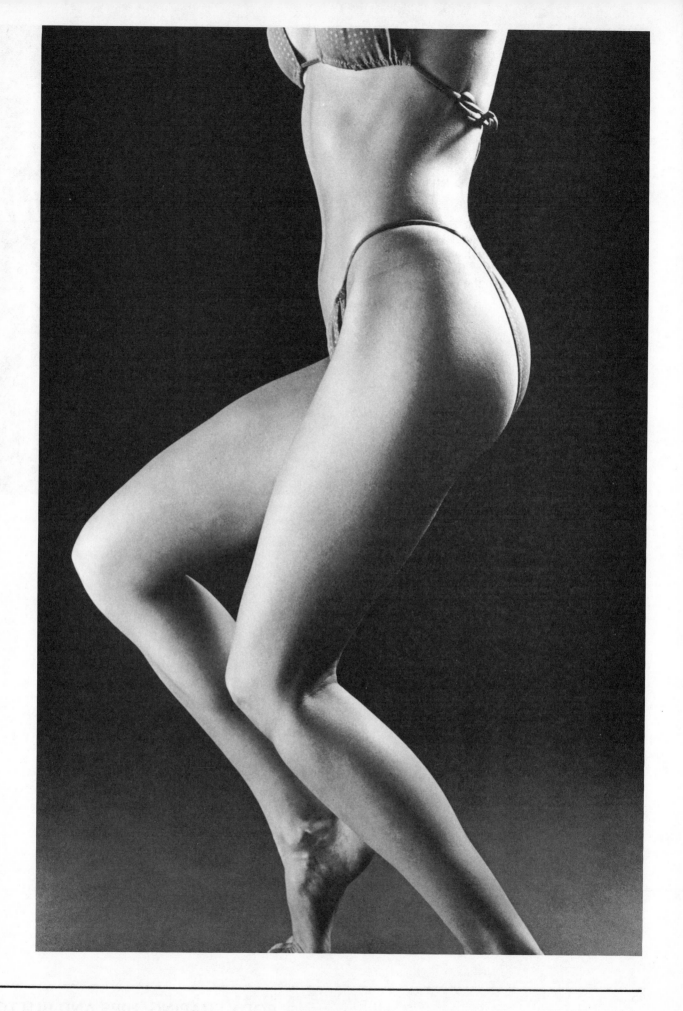

CHAPTER 5
THIGHS

Heavy thighs seem to be the most common figure problem for women. Upper thighs bulge, inner thighs sag, and back thighs become rippled.

Since women tend to store more fat directly under the skin around the thighs than men do, it is especially important that they keep the thigh muscles as strong as possible. Strong leg muscles will prevent much of the overlying fat and skin from sagging.

Anatomy of the Thigh

Some of the largest muscles of the body are found in the thigh. The quadriceps muscles are located on the front thigh. They cross both the knee and the hip joints. When these muscles contract, the leg extends and the hip joint flexes. On the back thigh are three muscles called hamstrings. The hamstrings also cross the knee and the hip joint. They bend the leg and extend the hip.

The inner thighs consist of five muscles of which the adductor magnus is the largest. The function of these muscles is to move the thighs from a spread-legged position to a knees-together position.

The woman who performs body-shaping exercise for the thighs in the recommended fashion should expect to see increased strength and muscle tone in less than a month. Firmer and more slender thighs are definitely a reality.

EXERCISE:
PARTNER LEG CURL

RATING: A
EQUIPMENT:
PARTNER AND
MEDIUM-SIZED
TOWEL

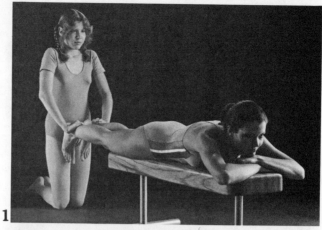

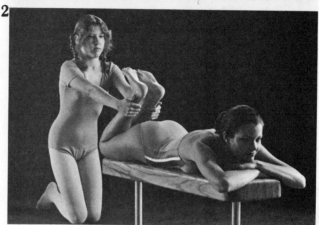

Starting Position: Lie face-down on a bench and position both knees just off the edge at the end. If needed, use a folded bath towel for padding.

Movement: Alternately bend and straighten the legs against the resistance provided by a partner. Continue until fatigued.

EXERCISE:
LEANING KNEE BEND

RATING: A
EQUIPMENT:
BARBELL

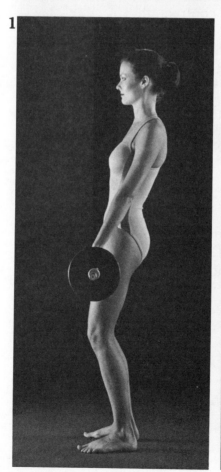

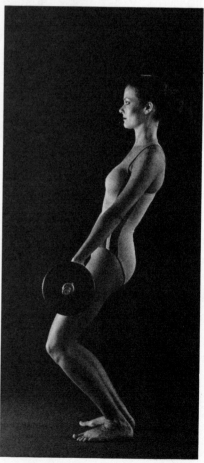

Starting Position: Grasp a barbell. Stand and place at arms' length against thighs. The feet should be shoulder-width apart.

Movement: Assume a leaning-back position. Slowly bend at the knees only and lower the body. The thighs and torso must be in line with one another. Return to the starting position and repeat.

Hint: In order to obtain the greatest possible range of movement, the heels must be elevated at least three inches.

EXERCISE:
ONE-LEGGED SQUAT

RATING: A
EQUIPMENT: CHAIR

Starting Position: Grasp the back of a chair with the right hand and hold the right leg in front of the body. Do not let the right foot touch the floor. Stand erect. Keep the foot flat if working the back is desired. Keep the heel elevated if working the calf is more preferable.

Movement: Slowly lower the upper body by bending the left knee and hip. Look straight ahead or slightly upward during the movement. Continue downward until the back of the left thigh comes into contact with the left calf. **Do not** bounce at the bottom of the movement. **Do not** relax at the bottom of the movement. Return smoothly to the starting position and repeat. Work the right leg in the same manner.

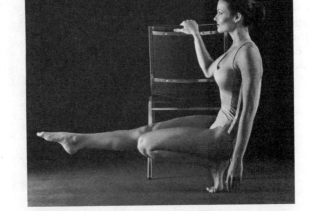

1
2

EXERCISE:
NEGATIVE-EMPHASIZED SQUAT WITH PARTNER

RATING: A
EQUIPMENT: PARTNER

Starting Position: Stand erect with the feet shoulder-width apart. From behind a partner places her hands on the squatter's shoulders.

Movement: As the knees bend the partner applies pressure downward. Very slow movements are called for in this exercise. At the bottom position, the pressure is removed and the squatter returns to the top position where the partner resumes the negative resistance.

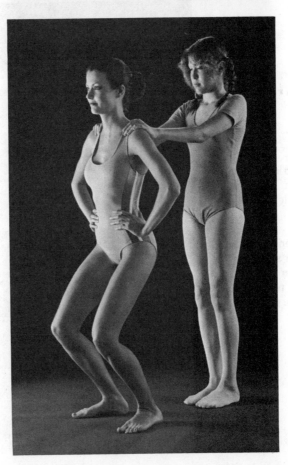

BODY SHAPING: THIGHS

EXERCISE:
CHAIR STEP-UP
WITH PLASTIC
BOTTLE

RATING: A
EQUIPMENT:
CHAIR AND
WATER-FILLED
PLASTIC BOTTLE

Starting Position: Stand erect with the left foot planted firmly in a straight-bottomed chair and the other on the floor. The bottle is held in one hand.

Movement: Slowly step up onto the chair, then step down with the same leg and up again until it is completely fatigued. Switch sides and step up with the other leg.

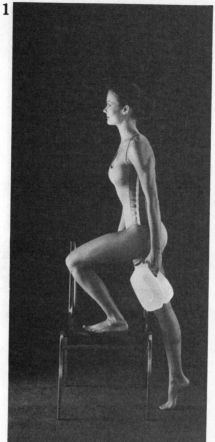
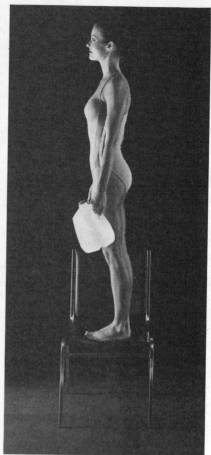

EXERCISE:
HIP ADDUCTION
WITH PARTNER

RATING: A
EQUIPMENT:
PARTNER

Starting Position: Sit on the floor facing a partner. Both should lean back, using the elbows for support. Keep the legs straight. Place the ankles outside the partner's ankles.

Movement: Squeeze the legs forcibly together against the partner's attempt to spread them. The partner provides both the positive and negative resistance, which is felt in the groin and inner thigh area. Repeat.

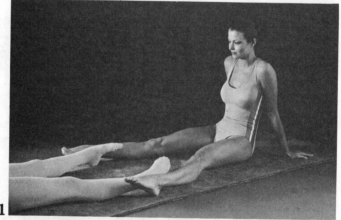
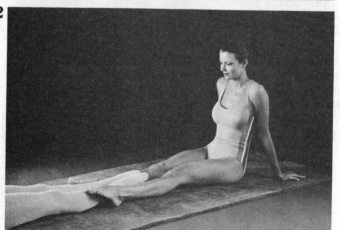

EXERCISE:
HIP ADDUCTION WITH PARTNER

RATING: A
EQUIPMENT: PARTNER

Starting Position: Sit on the floor facing a partner. Both should lean back, using the elbows for support. Keep the legs straight. Place the ankles inside the partner's ankles.

Movement: Spread the legs forcibly against the partner's squeezing resistance. The partner should allow positive and negative work of this spreading function. This is felt in the outer hips. Repeat until fatigued.

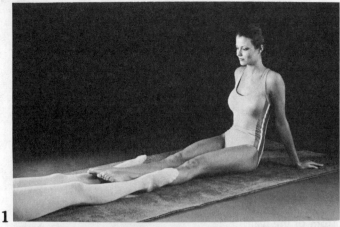

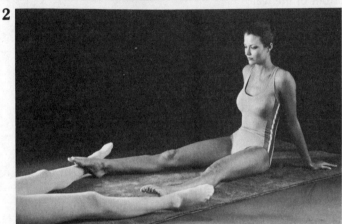

EXERCISE:
CHAIR STEP-UP

RATING: B
EQUIPMENT: CHAIR

Starting Position: Stand erect with the left foot planted firmly in a straight-bottomed chair and the other on the floor.

Movement: Slowly step up onto the chair, then step down with the same leg until it is completely fatigued. Switch sides and step up with the other leg.

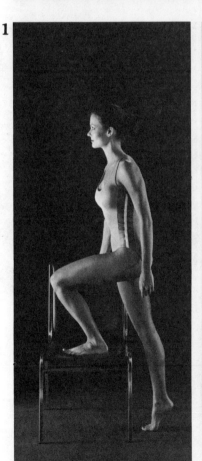

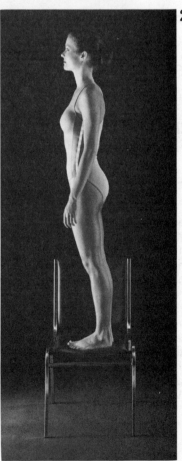

BODY SHAPING: THIGHS

EXERCISE:
WALL LEG
PRESS

RATING: B
EQUIPMENT:
SMOOTH WALL

Starting Position: Stand erect and lean back against a smooth, sturdy wall. Both heels should be approximately one-foot away from the wall, and shoulder-width apart. A cushion may be placed at the bottom of the wall.

Movement: Bend at the knees and slide the body down the wall. The object of the wall leg press is to descend as slowly as possible for one repetition. The movement gets more difficult as the body lowers. An adequate lowering time is from 30 to 60 seconds.

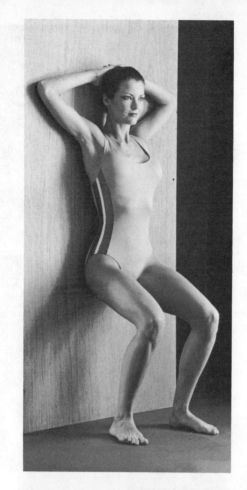

EXERCISE:
LUNGE WITH
PLASTIC
BOTTLES

RATING: B
EQUIPMENT:
WATER-FILLED
PLASTIC
BOTTLES

Starting Position: With plastic bottles at arms length to the sides, stand erect. Place the left foot in front of the right. The wider the feet are placed, the more stretch in the exercise.

Movement: Keeping the right leg straight, lower the body by bending the left leg at the knee. **Do not** relax at the bottom of the movement or bounce. The back should remain vertical as it moves forward. Straighten the left leg and repeat. When completed, switch to right leg.

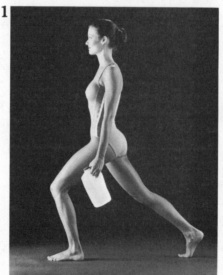

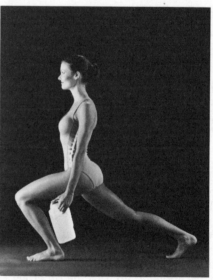

EXERCISE:
STRADDLE LIFT
WITH A
BARBELL

RATING: B
EQUIPMENT:
BARBELL

Starting Position: Straddle a barbell and grasp the bar in front and behind the body.

Movement: Lift the barbell and stand erect by straightening the legs slowly. Keep the head and shoulders up. Lower slowly and repeat.

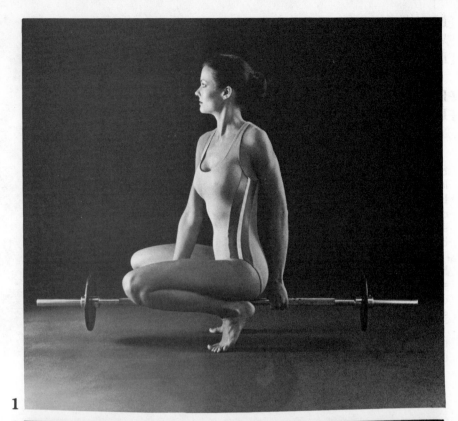

1

2

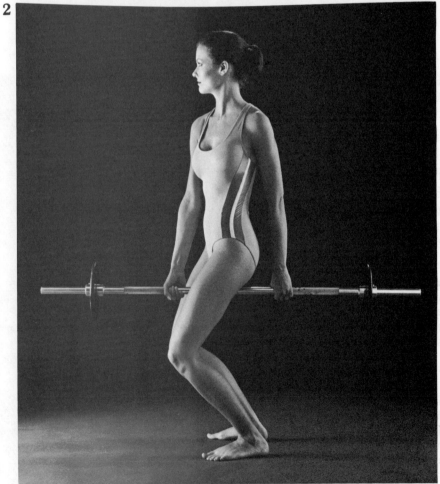

53

EXERCISE:
STIFF-LEGGED
DEADLIFT

RATING: B
EQUIPMENT:
BARBELL

Starting Position: Grasp the barbell.

Movement: Keep the arms straight, but bend the knees to lift the weight to the standing position: **Slowly** lower, then raise the load keeping **both** the arms and legs straight. Repeat until fatigued.

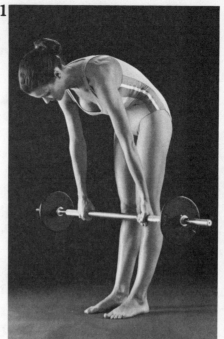

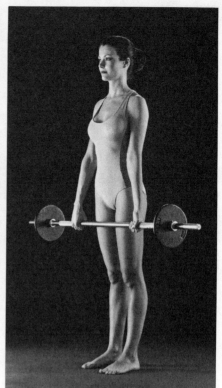

EXERCISE:
SQUAT

RATING: B
EQUIPMENT:
NONE

Starting Position: Stand erect with the heels flat. The feet should be shoulder-width apart.

Movement: Lower the body by bending the knees as far as possible. Keep the back vertical. Return to the starting position and repeat. **Do not** bounce or relax at the bottom of the movement.

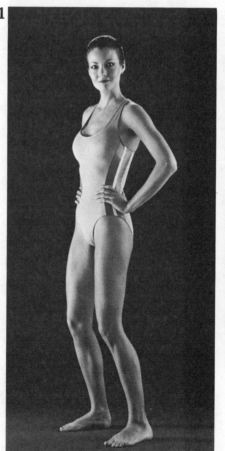

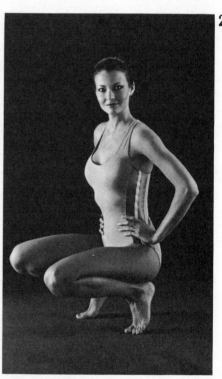

EXERCISE:
WIDE SQUAT

RATING: **B**
EQUIPMENT:
NONE

Starting Position: Place the feet twice shoulder-width apart and turn the toes outward. Stand erect with the heels flat. Rest the hands on the head.

Movement: Lower the body by bending the knees as far as possible. Keep the back vertical. Return to starting position and repeat. **Do not** bounce or relax at the bottom of the movement.

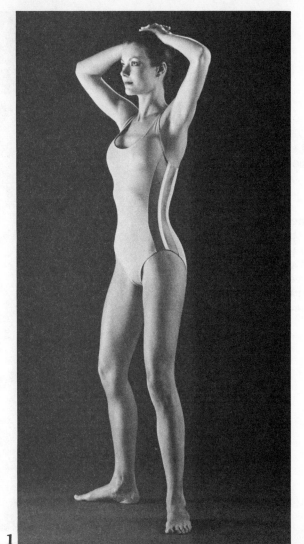

1

2

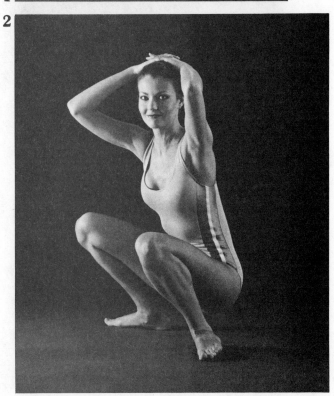

EXERCISE:
LUNGE

RATING: B
EQUIPMENT:
NONE

Starting Position: Stand erect. Place the left foot in front of the right. The wider the feet are placed, the more stretch in the exercise.

Movement: Keeping the right leg straight, lower the body by bending the left leg at the knee. **Do not** relax at the bottom of the movement or bounce. The back should remain vertical as it moves forward. Straighten the left leg and repeat. When completed, switch to right leg.

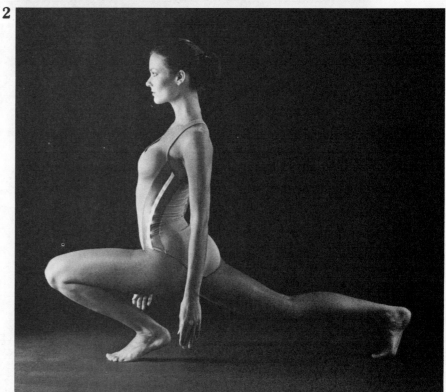

1

2

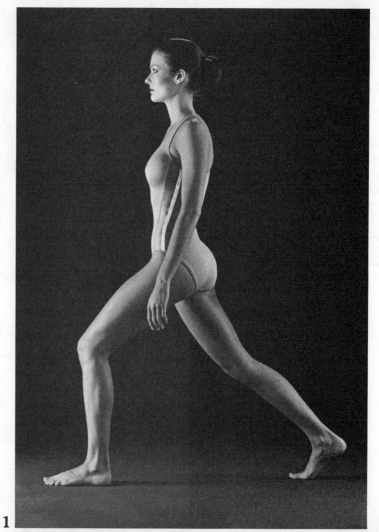

EXERCISE:
BENT-OVER
ONE-LEGGED
SQUAT

RATING: B
EQUIPMENT:
CHAIR

Starting position: Stand and face a straight chair. Bend at the hips and support the upper body with outstretched arms on the seat of the chair. Pick up the right foot and prevent it from touching the floor.

Movement: Slowly squat as low as possible with the left leg. **Do not** bounce or relax at the bottom of the movement. Return to the starting position and repeat. Then switch legs and squat with the other leg.

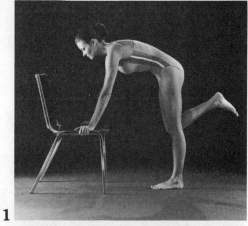

1

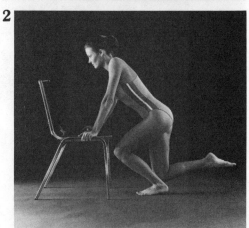

2

EXERCISE:
INNER THIGH
SQUEEZE

RATING: B
EQUIPMENT:
NONE

Starting Position: Sit on the floor with the legs in front of the body, knees bent, and the soles of the feet together. Reach between the knees and grasp just above the ankles with both hands. The elbows should be against the inner thighs.

Movement: Alternately squeeze and spread the knees against the resistance provided by the elbows. Perform slowly until the inner thighs are fatigued.

1

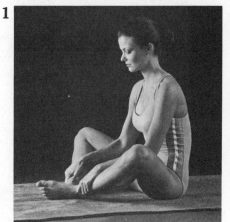

2

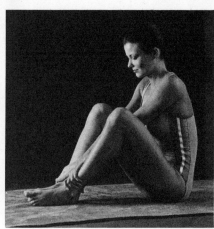

57

EXERCISE:
OUTER THIGH SQUEEZE

RATING: B
EQUIPMENT: NONE

Starting Position: Sit on the floor with the legs in front of the body, knees bent, and the soles of the feet together. Place the palms on the outer surface of the knees.

Movement: Alternately squeeze and spread the knees against the resistance provided by the hands. Perform slowly until fatigued.

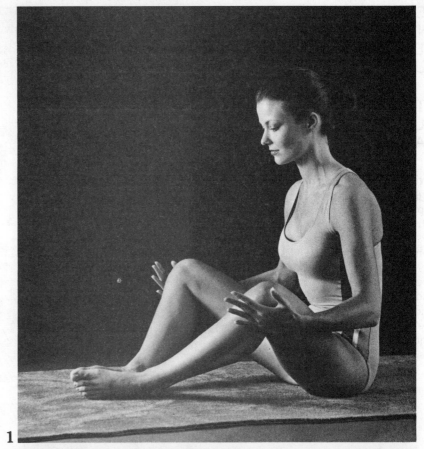

1

2

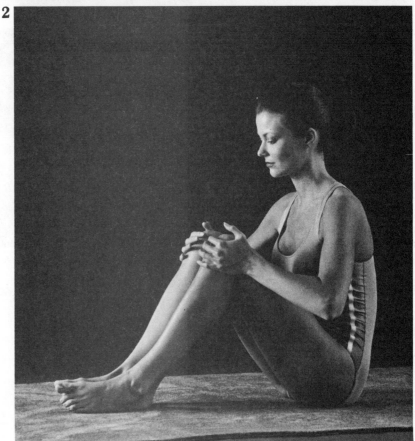

EXERCISE:
DOUBLE LEG
RAISE TO
SIDE

RATING: C
EQUIPMENT:
NONE

Starting Position: Lie on the right side with the right arm extended on the floor outward and upward from the head. The left elbow should touch the body with hand placed on the floor for balance.

Movement: With the knees and feet touching and the legs absolutely straight, raise them sideways as high as possible. Pause, slowly lower, and repeat. Reverse sides and do the movement with the left arm above the head and the right hand on the floor.

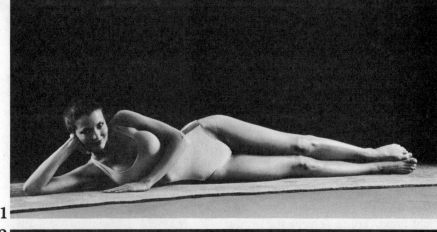

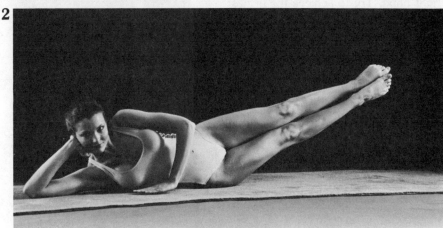

EXERCISE:
SIDE LEG
CIRCLE

RATING: C
EQUIPMENT:
NONE

Starting Position: Assume a crawling stance on the floor. Support the body on the hands, arms straight, and the right knee. The left leg should be straight and the foot suspended off the floor.

Movement: Slowly draw an imaginary circle with the left foot. This circular motion should be as large as possible. Keep the leg straight. Continue for one minute. Then switch legs.

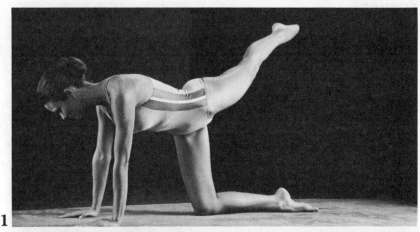

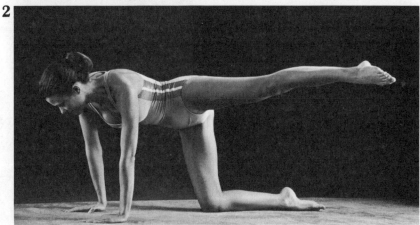

59

EXERCISE:
STANDING THIGH RAISE

RATING: C
EQUIPMENT: NONE

Starting position: Stand on the left leg.

Movement: Raise and lower the right thigh against resistance provided by right hand. Try to achieve the highest possible position with the thigh. Perform 8-12 repetitions with the right, then 8-12 with the left.

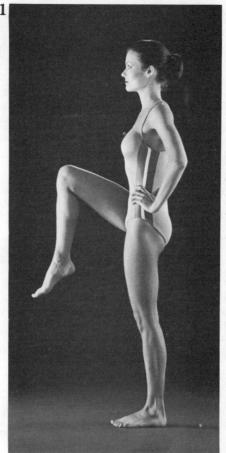
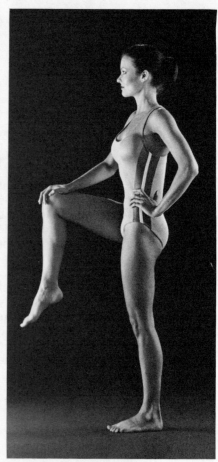

EXERCISE:
STANDING SIDE LEG RAISE

RATING: C
EQUIPMENT: CHAIR

Starting Position: Stand erect with the back of a chair to the right side of the body. For balance, grasp the chair with the right hand. Hold the left arm straight and out to the left side of the body.

Movement: Slowly raise the left leg laterally to meet the stationary left arm. Lower slowly and repeat. Switch sides to work the right leg.

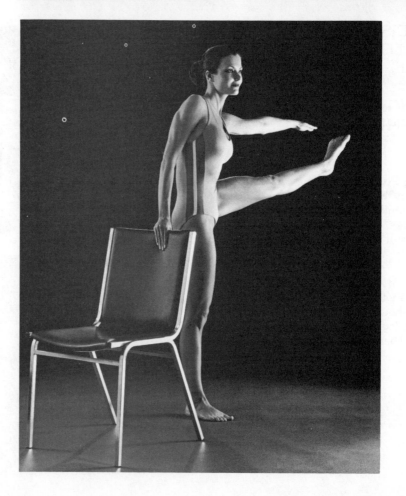

EXERCISE:
LYING SIDE
LEG RAISE

RATING: C
EQUIPMENT:
NONE

Starting Position: Lie on the right side of the body. Support the head with the right hand braced against the elbow. The legs should be straight and in line with the torso. The left leg should rest atop and along the right leg.

Movement: Keeping the left leg straight, raise it as high as possible. Lower slowly and repeat. Switch sides to work the right leg.

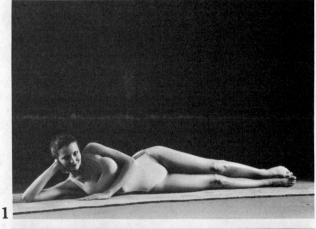

1

2

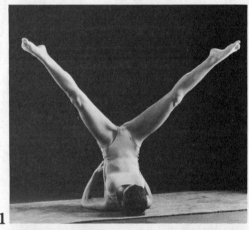

EXERCISE:
SHOULDER STAND
LEG SCISSOR

RATING: C
EQUIPMENT:
NONE

Starting Position: Perform a body stand on the floor with the shoulders and elbows. The chin should be on the chest, with the arms bent, the hands on the back of the rib cage, and the legs straight up. Keep the knees locked and the toes pointed.

Movement: Scissor the legs laterally, first front and then back for 8-12 slow repetitions.

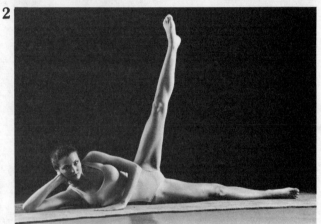

1

2

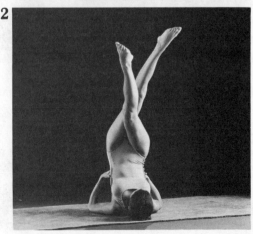

BODY SHAPING: THIGHS

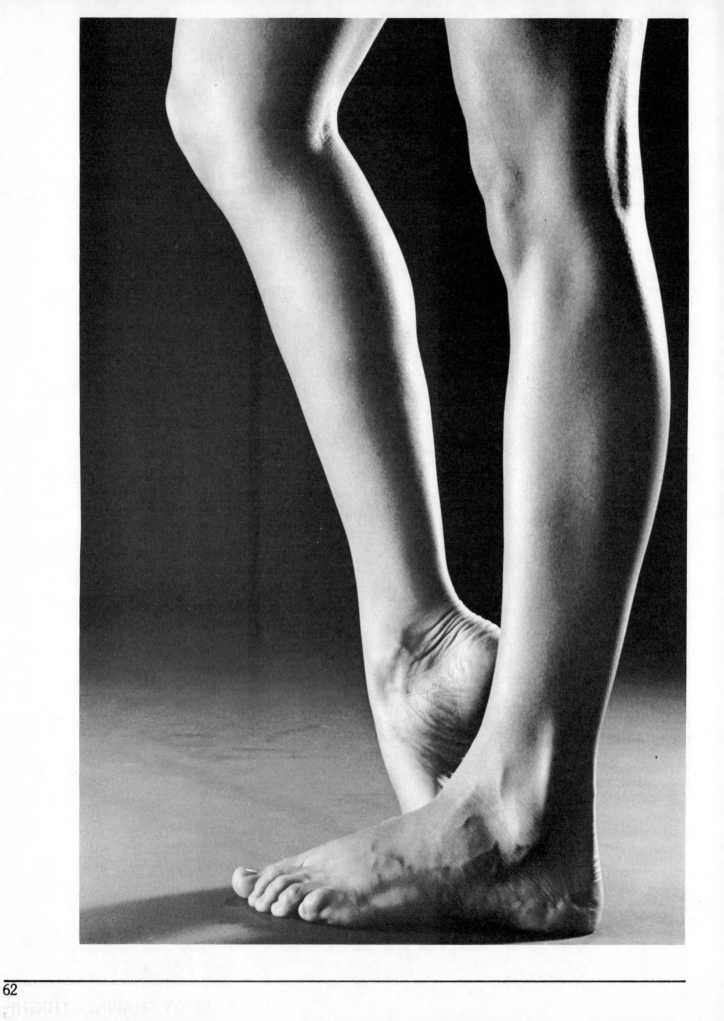

CHAPTER 6
CALVES

Few women worry about their calves. They should realize, however, that calves are just as important to attractive legs as slim thighs. Shapely calves can be some of the sexiest muscles of a woman's body. Just ask Juliet Prowse, the famous dancer and entertainer, who has been doing panty hose commercials on television for years. Because of her perfectly formed calves, she is admired by people all over the world.

There is another benefit to having strong, shapely calves. Exercising the calves positively affects the ankles. Strong and flexible ankles will help prevent injuries to this vulnerable area that active women frequently injure.

Anatomy of the Calf

The anatomy of the calf is fairly simple. The major muscle of the calf is the gastrocnemius, the U-shaped muscle at the rear of the lower leg. This muscle makes up most of the mass of the calf and performs the major function of lifting the body on the toes.

In additon to the gastrocnemius, there are several other muscles on the front and side areas of the calf. There are the tibialis group, the soleus, and the peroneus group. The function of these muscles is limited, consisting mainly of moving the foot up and down, with some side motion.

For best results, calf exercises should be performed immediately after the thighs are worked. Keeping the calves in proportion with the thighs is certain to beautify the feminine physique.

BODY SHAPING

EXERCISE:
ONE-LEGGED CALF
RAISE WITH
PLASTIC BOTTLE

RATING: A

EQUIPMENT:
MINIMUM THREE-INCH
BLOCK OR STAIR STEP,
PLASTIC BOTTLE,
AND CHAIR

Starting Position: Place the ball of the left foot on the edge of a block or stair step. Lock the knee and suspend the other foot. Grasp a water-filled bottle in one hand and balance the body with the other by grasping a chair or stair rail.

Movement: While the knee remains locked, raise the heel as high as possible, then lower slowly to a deep stretch. Repeat until fatigued. Follow the same procedure for the right calf.

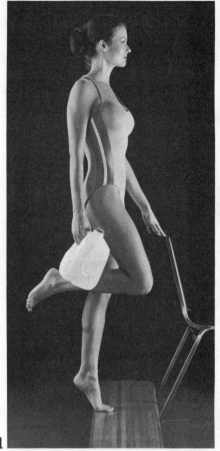

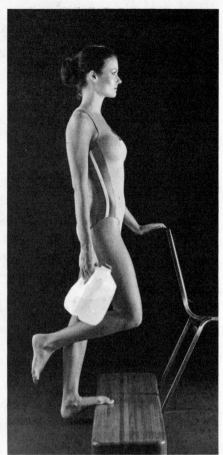

EXERCISE:
ONE-LEGGED
CALF RAISE

RATING: A

EQUIPMENT:
MINIMUM THREE-INCH
BLOCK OR STAIR
STEP AND CHAIR

Starting Position: Place the ball of the left foot on the edge of a block or stair step. Lock the knees and suspend the other foot. Balance the body by grasping a chair or stair rail.

Movement: While the knee remains locked, raise the heel as high as possible, then lower slowly to a deep stretch. Repeat until fatigued. Follow the same procedure for the right calf.

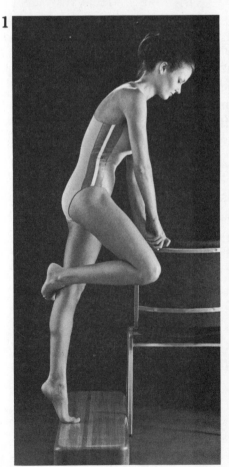

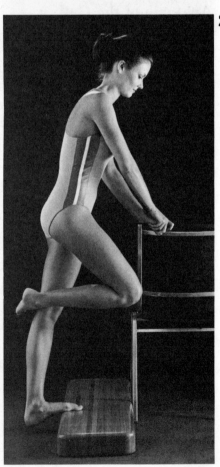

EXERCISE:
PARTNER FOOT
FLEXION

RATING: A
EQUIPMENT:
PARTNER AND
BENCH

Starting Position: Sit on a bench with the legs straight.

Movement: Have a partner pull the tops of the feet away from the knee. Raise the foot toward the knee against the partner's resistance. Repeat.

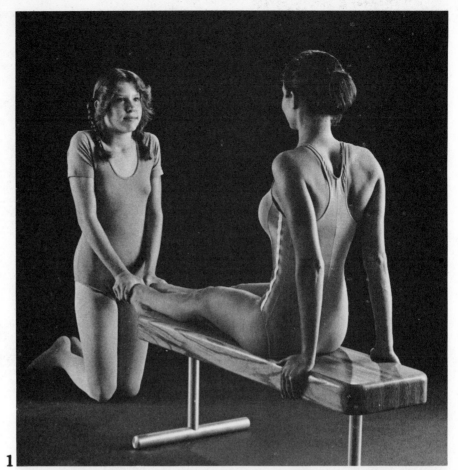

1

2

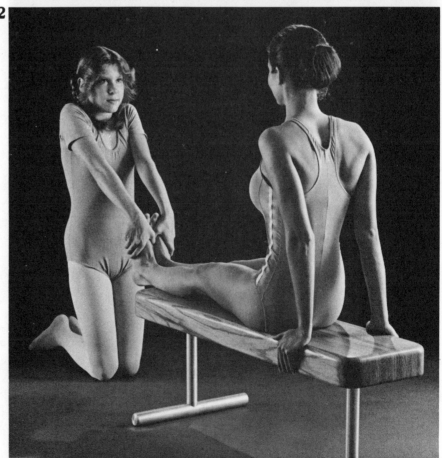

BODY SHAPING: CALVES

EXERCISE:
CALF RAISE

RATING: B

EQUIPMENT:
MINIMUM THREE-INCH
BLOCK OR STAIR STEP
AND CHAIR

Starting Position: Place the balls of
both feet on the edge of a block or stair
step. Lock the knees. Balance the body
by grasping a chair or stair rail.

Movement: While the knees remain
locked raise both heels as high as
possible, then lower slowly to a deep
stretch. Repeat until fatigued.

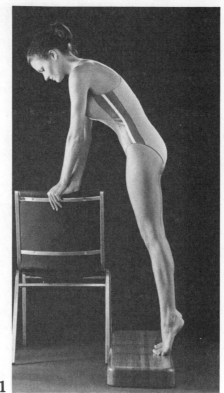

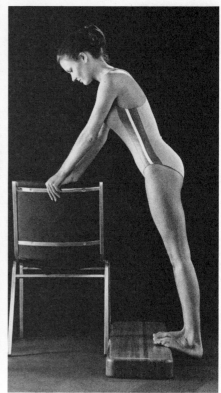

1

2

EXERCISE:
OUTSIDE ANKLE
STRENGTHENING AGAINST
A DOOR

RATING: B

EQUIPMENT:
CHAIR AND
SWINGING DOOR

Starting Position: Sit in a chair next to
the edge of an open door. Move door on
the outside of the right foot. The right
arm provides the resistance.

Movement: The knee and heel should
remain stationary as the side of the foot
moves from left to right against the
door. The outside of the left ankle is
exercised in the same fashion.

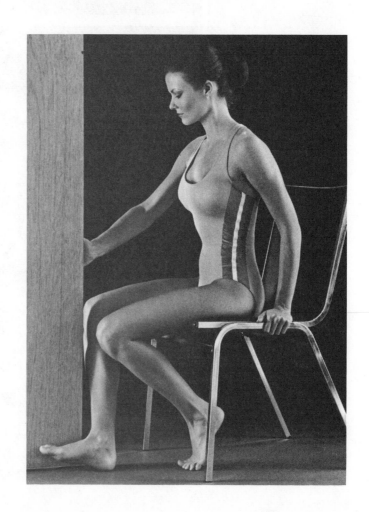

EXERCISE:
INSIDE ANKLE STRENGTHENING AGAINST A DOOR

RATING: B
EQUIPMENT:
CHAIR AND SWINGING DOOR

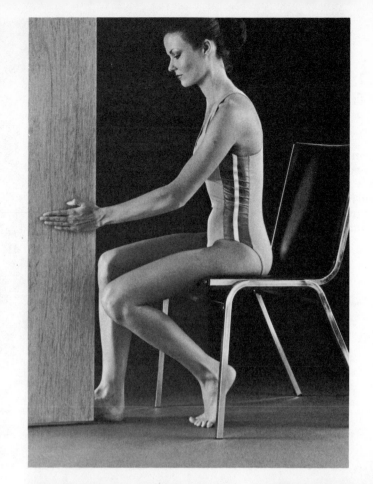

Starting Position: Sit in a chair next to the edge of an open door. Place the side of the right foot on the side of the door. Resistance is provided by the left arm against the door.

Movement: The knee and heel should remain stationary as the ball of the foot moves from right to left against the door. The inside of the other ankle is worked in the same fashion.

EXERCISE:
SEATED CALF RAISE

RATING: B
EQUIPMENT:
CHAIR AND MINIMUM THREE-INCH BLOCK OR STAIR STEP

Starting Position: Sit in a chair. Place the balls of both feet on the edge of a block or stair step located directly in front of the chair.

Movement: Raise the heels as high as possible. Pause, then lower slowly to a deep stretch, and repeat.

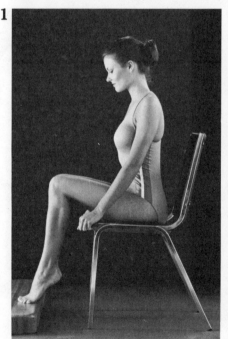

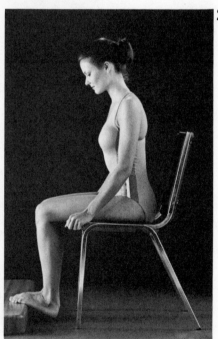

EXERCISE:
TOE CURL

RATING: B
EQUIPMENT:
CHAIR

Starting Position: Sit erect with the feet flat on the floor.

Movement: Try to raise the toes as high as possible without moving the heels. Pause. Return and repeat.

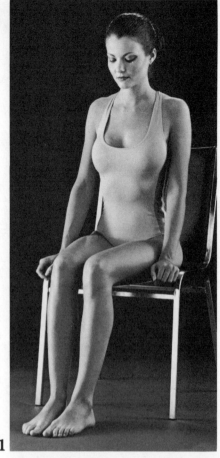

1

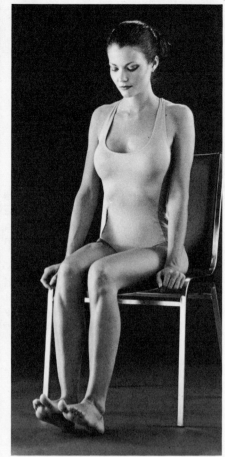

2

EXERCISE:
BENT-OVER
CALF RAISE

RATING: B
EQUIPMENT:
MINIMUM THREE-INCH
BLOCK OR STAIR STEP
AND CHAIR

Starting Position: Place the balls of both feet on the edge of a block or stair step. Lean over and support the upper body with outstretched arms or the seat of a chair. Lock the knees.

Movement: Raise the heels as high as possible. Pause, then lower slowly to a deep stretch. Repeat.

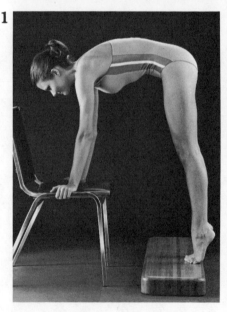

1

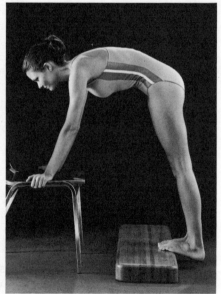

2

EXERCISE:
TOE SPREAD

RATING: C
EQUIPMENT:
CHAIR

Starting Position: Sit erect with the feet flat on the floor.

Movement: Spread the toes as the front of the foot presses downward toward the floor. Release. Repeat until fatigued.

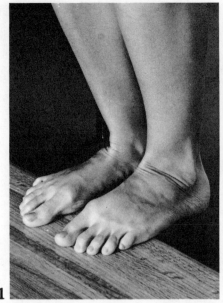

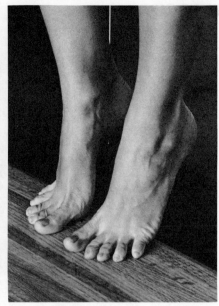

EXERCISE:
ANKLE CIRCLE

RATING: C
EQUIPMENT:
CHAIR

Starting Position: Sit in a chair and cross the left leg over the right.

Movement: Perform circular motions with the left foot. Repeat for one minute. Change feet.

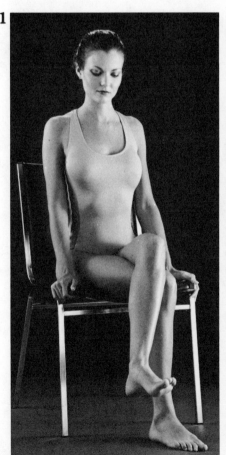

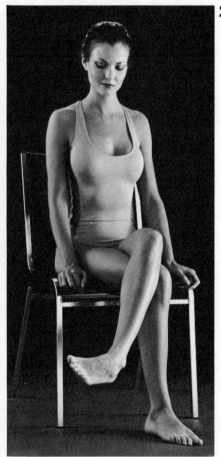

BODY SHAPING: CALVES

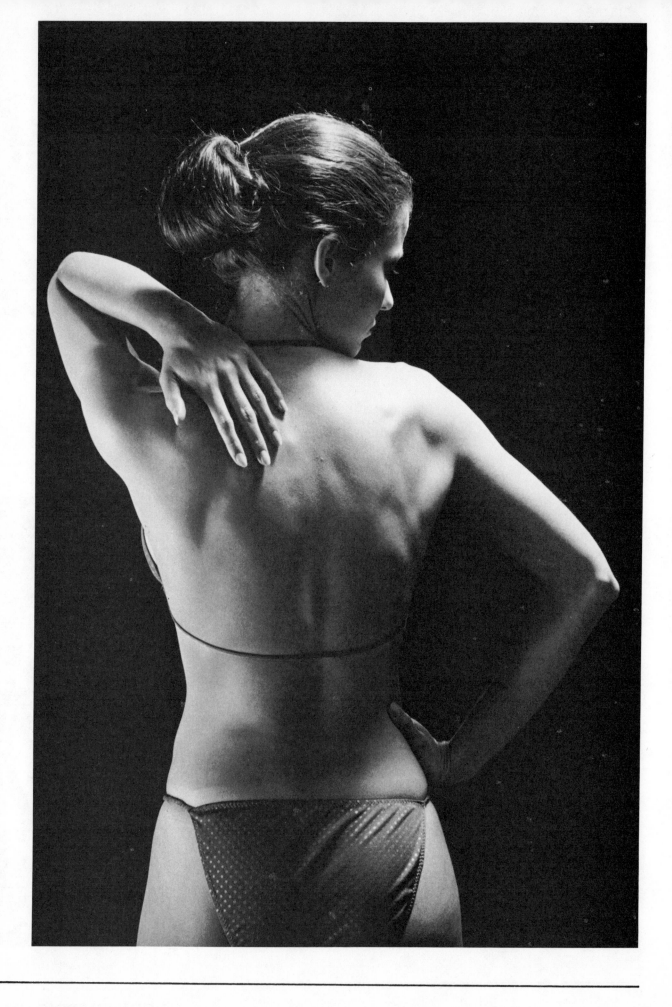

CHAPTER 7
BACK

Raquel Welch was recently asked what she considered the most outstanding part of her body. "It's my back," she said to the amazed reporter.

Some people might disagree with Raquel's choice. Most women's fashions emphasize long legs and shapely bosoms. But Raquel's selection certainly makes sense from a physiological point of view.

The largest and strongest muscle of the upper body is on the back. This muscle has been appropriately named latissimus dorsi, which means "widest of the back."

Strong, shapely latissimus muscles give the much-admired "V" shape to the male physique. They also add sex appeal to the female figure. Strong musculature in the back supports the posture, carriage, and gait, all of which give the look of poise and confidence.

Performance in numerous sports depends on the contraction of the latissimus and several other back muscles. Throwing, hitting, swimming, skiing, and all activities that involve pulling movements, activate the muscles of the back.

Anatomy of the Back

The strongest muscle of the back is the latissimus dorsi. These muscles join the lower part of the spine and sweep up to the armpit where they are inserted into the upper arm bone. When the latissimus dorsi muscles contract, they pull the upper arms from an overhead position down and around the shoulder axes. This rotational movement can take place with the upper arms in front of the body or on the sides of the body.

Several smaller back muscles also assist the latissimus in moving the upper arms. The most important of these muscles is the teres major.

The other large back muscle, the trapezius, plays an important role in correct posture. The trapezius is a flat triangular muscle that extends from the base of the skull across the width of the shoulders and comes to a tapering point half way down the spinal column. The most important of its functions is to elevate or shrug the shoulders. Strong trapezius muscles help support the head, shoulders, and spine.

Exercises for the large back muscles will be concerned with rotational movements of the upper arms and shrugging of the shoulders.

In addition to the impressive latissimus and trapezius muscles, another area of the back is of vital importance – the lower back. This part of the back is the foundation of the entire body. With insufficient lower back strength, a woman is limited in the strength she can develop in her upper and lower body.

Exercising the entire back, the wise woman will not neglect her back muscles in her quest for a strong, shapely body. Raquel Welch's beautiful back did not just happen. It is a result of proper exercise.

BODY SHAPING

EXERCISE:
CHINUP

RATING: A
EQUIPMENT:
HORIZONTAL BAR

Starting Position: Grasp the horizontal bar with the palms facing the body. Hang.

Movement: Pull the body upward so that the chin is over the bar. Pause. Slowly lower the body to the starting position and repeat.

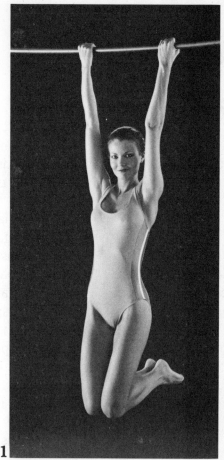

1

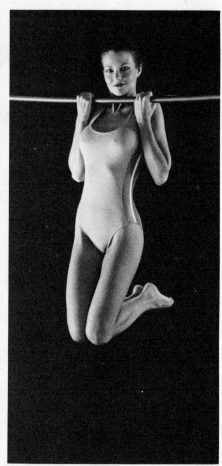

2

EXERCISE:
BENT-ARMED PULLOVER WITH PLASTIC BOTTLES

RATING: A
EQUIPMENT:
TWO WATER-FILLED PLASTIC BOTTLES AND BENCH

Starting Position: Lie face-up on a bench. The hands should be extended over the end and the feet should be hooked around the legs of the bench. Hold the plastic bottles over the shoulders in a bent-armed position.

Movement: Lower the weight toward the floor letting it come as close as possible to the forehead. Stretch in the bottom position. Return to the over-the-shoulder position and repeat.

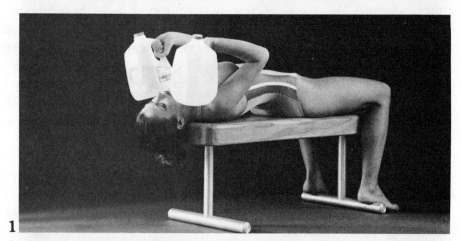

1

2

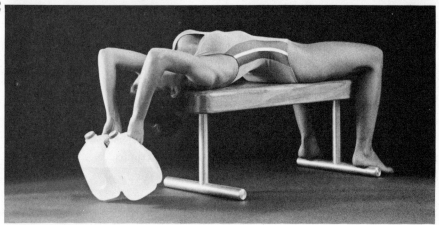

EXERCISE:
STIFF-LEGGED
DEADLIFT

RATING: A
EQUIPMENT:
BARBELL OR TWO
WATER-FILLED
PLASTIC BOTTLES

Starting Position: Grasp a barbell or a water-filled bottle in each hand.

Movement: Keep the arms straight, but bend the knees to lift the weight to the standing position. **Slowly** lower, then raise the load keeping the arms and legs straight. Repeat until fatigued.

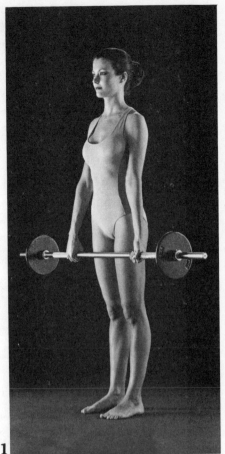

1

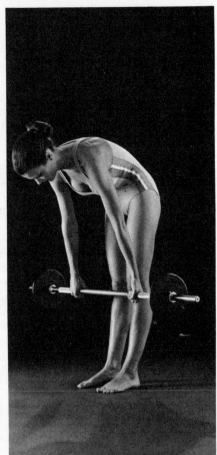

2

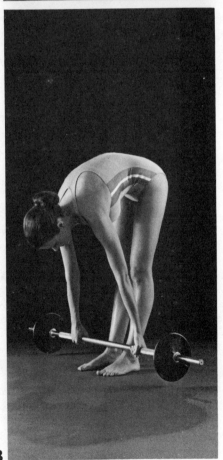

3

BODY SHAPING: BACK

EXERCISE:
STRAIGHT-ARMED PULLOVER WITH CANS

RATING: A
EQUIPMENT:
TWO UNOPENED CANS

Starting Position: Lie face-up on a bench. The head should be extended over the end and the feet should be on the floor. Hold the cans over the chest in a straight-armed position.

Movement: Take a deep breath, lower the weight behind the head and return to the over-the-chest position. It is important to keep the arms straight during the movement and to emphasize the stretching of the torso when the weight is behind the head.

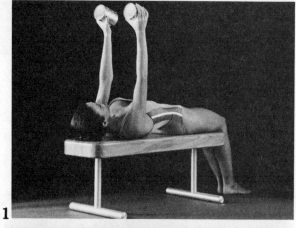

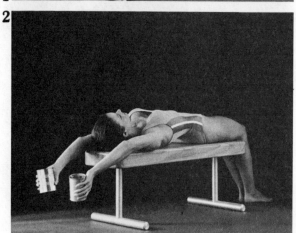

EXERCISE:
SHOULDER SHRUG WITH PLASTIC BOTTLES

RATING: A
EQUIPMENT:
TWO WATER-FILLED PLASTIC BOTTLES

Starting Position: Grasp the bottles and stand.

Movement: Keeping the arms straight, smoothly shrug the shoulders as high as possible. Pause in the top position. Slowly lower and repeat.

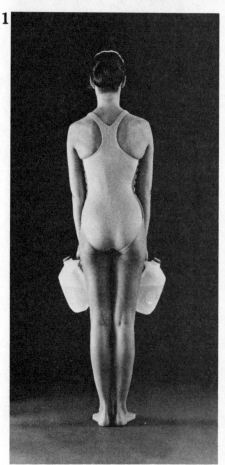

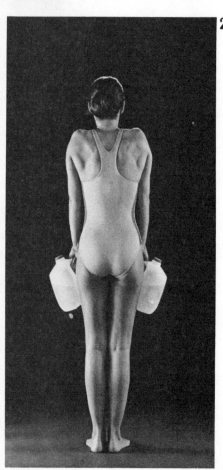

EXERCISE:
LYING CHINUP

RATING: B

EQUIPMENT:
BROOM HANDLE AND
TWO CHAIRS

Starting Position: Span an approximate two-foot distance between two chairs with the broom handle across the backs. Position the upper body under the broom handle. Grasp the handle with the palms facing the body.

Movement: Pull the chest to the broom handle. Pause and then lower slowly. Keep the body straight. Only the heels should touch the floor. If too difficult, allow the body to bend slightly as it is lifted, then keep it straight and rigid as it is lowered.

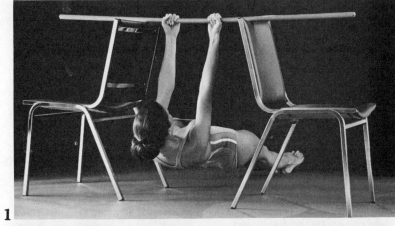

1

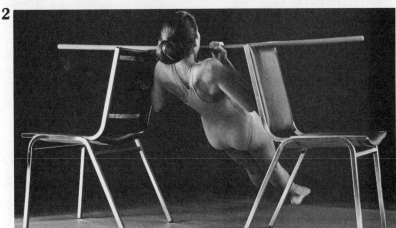

2

EXERCISE:
BENT-OVER ROW WITH
PLASTIC BOTTLES

RATING: B

EQUIPMENT:
TWO WATER-FILLED
PLASTIC BOTTLES

Starting Position: In a bent-over position, grasp two plastic bottles. The torso should be parallel with the floor.

Movement: Pull the hands upward until they touch the lower chest area. Pause. Slowly return to the starting position and repeat.

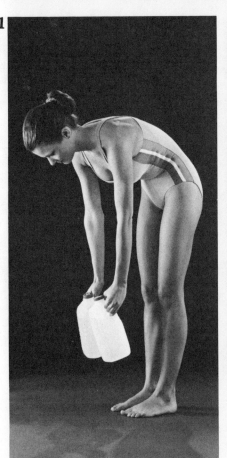

1

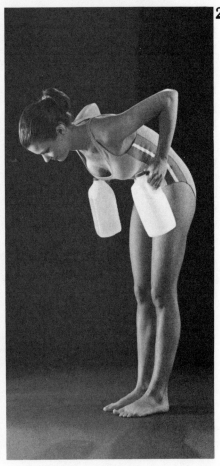

2

BODY SHAPING: BACK

EXERCISE:
BENT-OVER ROW

RATING: B
EQUIPMENT:
TWO UNOPENED CANS

Starting Position: In a bent-over position, grasp two cans. The torso should be parallel with the floor.

Movement: Pull the hands upward until they touch the lower chest area. Pause. Slowly return to the beginning position and repeat.

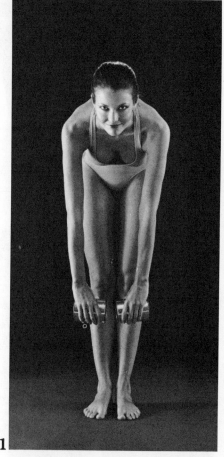

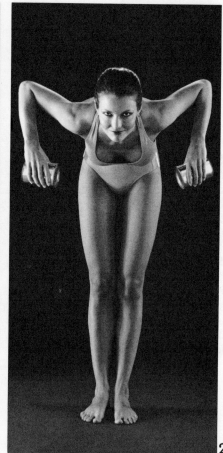

EXERCISE:
BACK HYPEREXTENSION
WITH A PARTNER

RATING: B
EQUIPMENT:
PARTNER AND BENCH

Starting Position: Lie face-down, length-wise on a bench. Support the lower half of the body by having the navel coincide with the edge of the bench. A partner should hold the legs and feet down.

Movement: Alternately raise and lower the torso keeping the hands behind the head. Repeat.

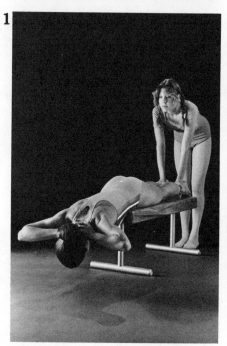

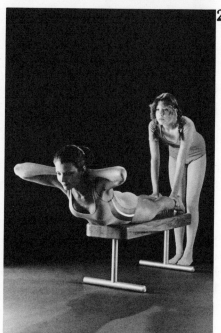

EXERCISE:
BACK HYPEREXTENSION AND REVERSE LEG RAISE

RATING: B

EQUIPMENT: NONE

Starting Position: Lie face-down on the floor. The hands should be interlaced behind the head with the body in a straight line.

Movement: Keeping the legs straight, attempt to arch the back slowly in such a way as to raise the feet and the upper body as high as possible off the floor. Pause in the raised position. Lower and repeat.

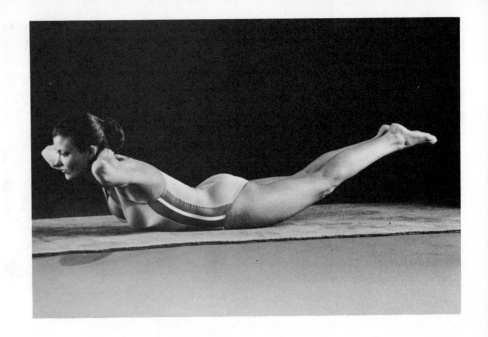

EXERCISE:
BENT-OVER LATERAL RAISE WITH CANS

RATING: B

EQUIPMENT: TWO UNOPENED CANS

Starting Position: Grasp a can in each hand. Bend over until the torso is parallel with the floor and the arms are hanging.

Movement: Keeping the arms straight, raise the cans outward and upward as far as possible. Pause. Slowly return to the starting position and repeat.

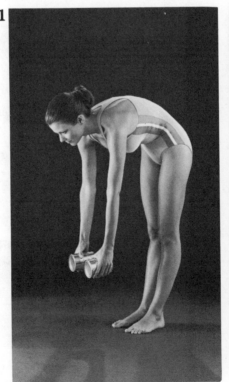

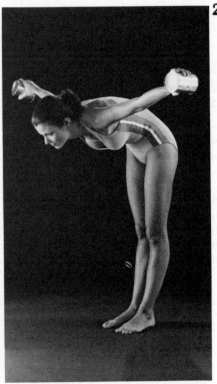

EXERCISE:
LATERAL RAISE WITH CANS

RATING: B
EQUIPMENT:
TWO OPENED CANS

Starting Position: Stand erect with a can in each hand. The arms should be by the sides of the body.

Movement: Keeping the arms straight, slowly raise the cans laterally to shoulder height. Pause. Lower and repeat.

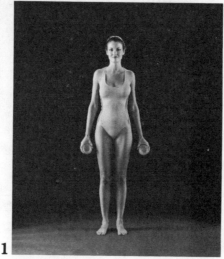

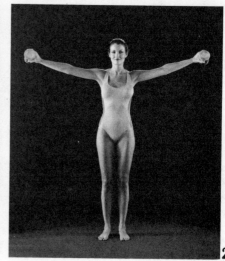

EXERCISE:
REVERSE LEG RAISE

RATING: C
EQUIPMENT:
NONE

Starting Position: Lie face-down on the floor. The hands should be by the hips.

Movement: Lift both legs backward as far as possible. Pause briefly at the highest position and strongly squeeze the buttocks together. Return the legs to the floor and repeat.

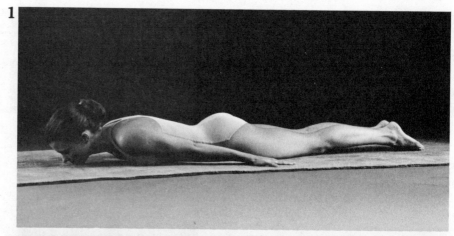

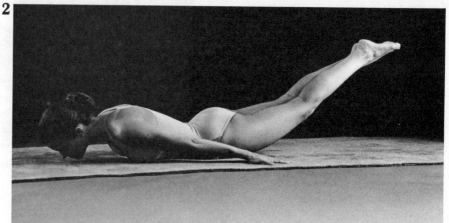

EXERCISE:
BACK HYPEREXTENSION

RATING: C
EQUIPMENT:
NONE

Starting Position: Lie face-down on the floor with entire body in a straight line. Interlace the hands behind the head.

Movement: Maintaining the legs firmly on the floor, attempt to raise the upper body slowly as high as possible. Pause. Lower and repeat.

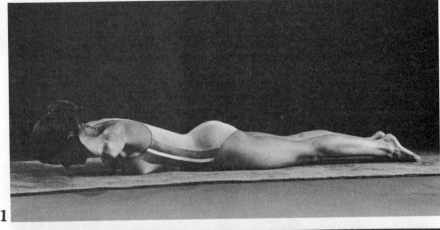

1

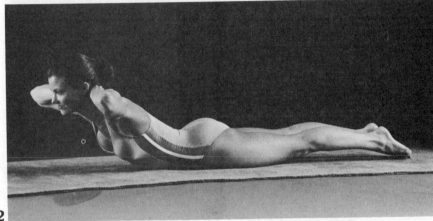

2

EXERCISE:
BENT-OVER SHRUG WITH PLASTIC BOTTLES

RATING: C
EQUIPMENT:
TWO WATER-FILLED PLASTIC BOTTLES

Starting Position: Grasp the bottles and hold at arms' length with legs straight and torso horizontal.

Movement: Lift the shoulders, pause, and lower. Do not allow the arms to bend. Repeat.

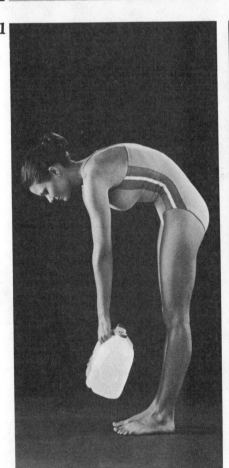

1

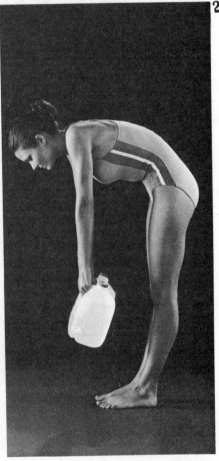

2

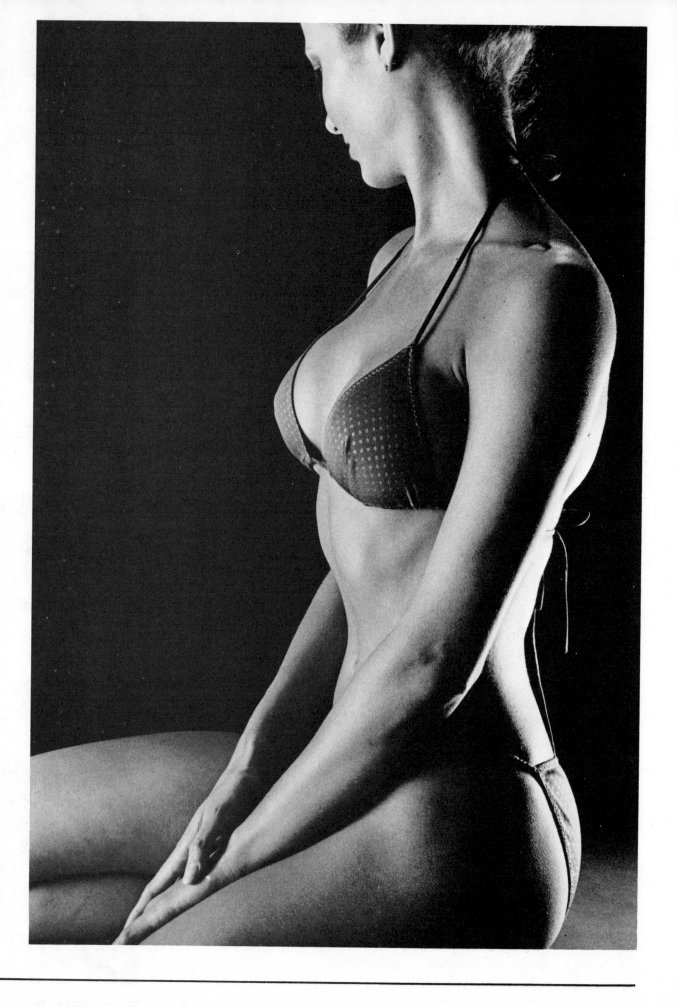

CHAPTER 8
BUST

"INSTANT INCHES ON THE BUST — 2 inches the first day, 3 inches the first week! Already a rumble is starting from the west to east about this startling innovation...about the bust developer everbody said could never be perfected..."

    -- From a recent advertisement in a popular woman's magazine

The girl on the left in the magazine advertisement looks rather pale, plain, and depressed.

The girl on the right in the same advertisement flashes a broad smile, framed by golden curls. She is radiant, confident, and the owner of a chest her brief sweater can barely contain.

Much to the reader's surprise , the model on the left and the model on the right are the same girl. The only difference is that the photographs were taken a mere four days apart.

How could such a plain Jane transform herself into every man's dream of a Scandinavian beauty queen between Monday and Friday? She simply gained "three beautiful inches" on her bust using the advertised exercise device.

Similar advertisements appear in numerous national magazines every month. A full page promotion in one magazine alone costs $13,000. In view of the cost of such advertising, the promoters must be pleased with the orders. A recent advertisement, in fact, boasted that it had sold four million bust developers at $9.95 each. That adds up to $40 million. Not bad for a product that is nothing more than two, five-inch circular pieces of plastic with a hinge at one end and a spring in the middle! The entire device is mass manufactured for about 32 cents each.

Turning a profit, however, should not be taken as an indication of the product's effectiveness.

Anyone who has studied human anatomy and exercise physiology knows that there is no muscle located in the female breast. Proper exercise may enlarge the latissimus dorsi muscles of the back and the pectoral muscles underlying the breasts, producing a slightly increased chest measurement. But growth of the breasts themselves is influenced by hormones that are released during puberty and pregnancy. Regardless of what advertisers print in women's magazines, there is no known exercise device that can improve the size of the female breast.

What the promoters fail to tell their female readers is that an effective make-up job combined with "trick" photography can appear to change a person's looks.

In the typical "before" picture, the model is facing straight into the camera, wearing a troubled half-smile. Her hair looks as if it has seen neither shampoo nor comb in a week. The black-and-white picture is unevenly lit, so any cleavage that might exist fades into the white of the halter top she is wearing.

In the "after" picture, the model is photographed at an angle. Her hair is cleaned and curled, her smile is full, and her make-up gives her a more vibrant look. The picture is professionally lit, with shading in all the proper places, especially down what has now become an incredible amount of cleavage.

The model has been girded into a tighter sweater, which, while maintaining the U-shaped neckline, is not a halter. As the garment attaches in front, the breasts are pushed up and together. Combine all of the above with super posture, a push-up bra, and the promoters have "instant inches." The entire process takes not a week, but less than an hour!

Anatomy of the Chest

Although the female breast can not be radically changed by exercise, numerous muscles of the chest can be strengthened in a short period of time. This strengthening will not only enhance appearance, but improve performance in many sports that involve torso muscles.

The pectoralis major is the most important muscle of the chest. One end is attached to the sternum and the other to the front of the upper arm. When the pectorals contract, they move the upper arms across the body. The male and female muscular structures are basically the same.

A woman, however, develops breasts in order to supply milk to the newborn infant. While the breasts are attached to the pectoralis major muscles, they are not composed of muscle tissue. Breasts are composed of fatty tissue, milk glands, connective tissue, and blood vessels. The only muscle in the female breast is a small involuntary one that is located in the erectile portion of the nipple and it has no potential for development.

Nothing can be done to increase the size of the female breast, outside of hormone drugs, silicone injections, or a large increase or decrease in body fat. Proper exercise, however, can definitely expand and increase the strength and tone of the underlying and surrounding muscle structures. As a result, the breasts will become firmer so they protrude more or are carried higher on the chest. Loose skin will also become tauter from proper exercise, and posture will be improved. A woman's bustline will take on new shape and contours as a result of improved tone and strength in the chest muscles.

EXERCISE:
STANDING CHAIR DIP

RATING: A
EQUIPMENT:
TWO CHAIRS

Starting Position: Face two chairs away from each other. Stand between them. Support the body on straightened arms against the backs of the chairs. Bend the legs at the knees.

Movement: Slowly lower the body by bending the arms. Stretch in the lowest position and smoothly return to the top. Repeat.

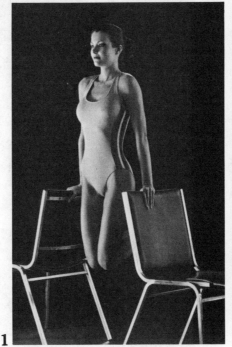

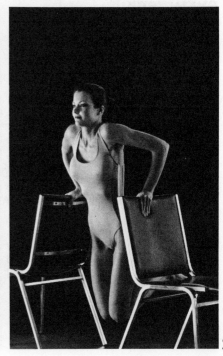

EXERCISE:
NEGATIVE CHAIR DIP

RATING: A
EQUIPMENT:
TWO CHAIRS

Starting Position: Face two chairs away from each other. Stand between them. Support the body on straightened arms against the backs of the chairs.

Movement: Slowly lower the body, then quickly stand to the straight-armed position and repeat until fatigued. If the arms cannot support the entire bodyweight at first, it is acceptable to cheat a little with assistance from the legs.

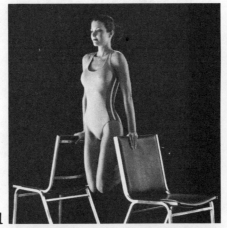

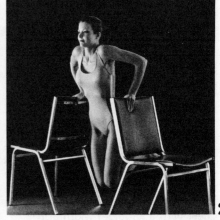

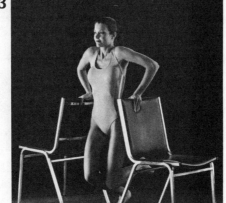

BODY SHAPING: BUST

EXERCISE:
BENCH PRESS
WITH BARBELL

RATING: A
EQUIPMENT:
BARBELL AND BENCH

Starting Position: For best results, it is necessary to have a bench with an attached barbell rack. In a face-up position, lift the barbell from the rack and bring it over the chest.

Movement: Lower the barbell slowly to the chest and immediately press it to the straight-arm position. Repeat until fatigued.

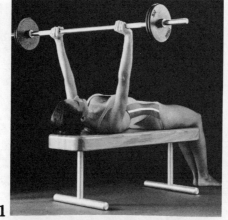

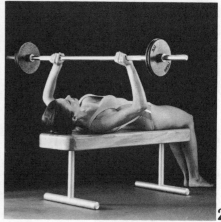

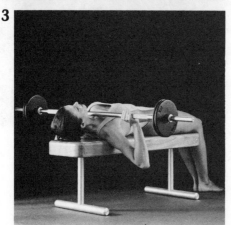

EXERCISE:
BENT-ARMED PULLOVER
WITH BARBELL

RATING: A
EQUIPMENT:
BARBELL AND BENCH

Starting Position: Lie face-up on a bench. The head should be extended over the end and the feet should be secured around the legs of the bench. The barbell should be held across the chest with a shoulder-width grip.

Movement: Lower the bar toward the floor letting it come as close as possible to the chin and forehead. Stretch in the bottom position. Return to the chest and repeat.

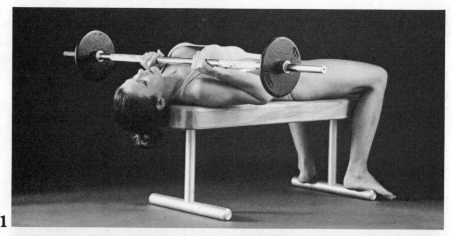

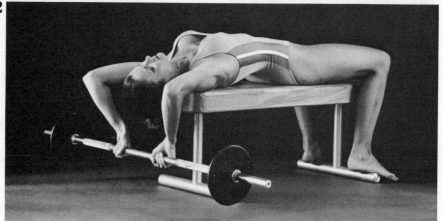

EXERCISE:
BENT-ARMED LATERAL RAISE WITH DUMBBELLS

RATING: A
EQUIPMENT:
DUMBBELLS AND BENCH

Starting Position: While seated on a narrow bench, grasp a dumbbell in each hand and bring them to rest on the thighs. Lie back on the bench and at the same time straighten the arms over the chest.

Movement: With the dumbbells over the chest, bend the arms and lower the dumbbells in a circular fashion to the sides of the chest. Stretch and return to the top position. It is important to keep the elbows wide on this exercise. Repeat.

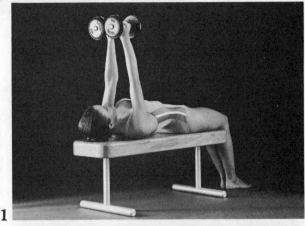
1

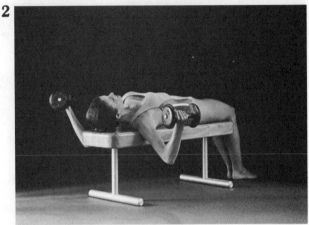
2

EXERCISE:
PUSHUP BETWEEN CHAIRS

RATING A
EQUIPMENT:
TWO CHAIRS

Starting Position: Position two chairs so that they face each other and their edges are shoulder-width apart. Place each hand on one of the chair seats. Hold the body straight and rigid as it is supported on the hands and toes.

Movement: Slowly push the body to arms' length and lower. Repeat.

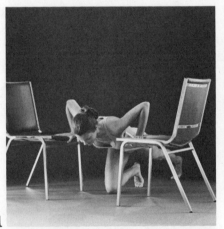
1

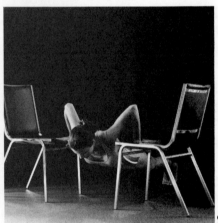
2

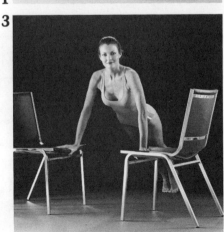
3

BODY SHAPING: BUST

EXERCISE:
BENT-ARM PULLOVER WITH PLASTIC BOTTLES

RATING: A
EQUIPMENT:
TWO WATER-FILLED PLASTIC BOTTLES AND BENCH

Starting Position: Lie face-up on a bench. The hands should be extended over the end and the feet should be secured around the legs of the bench. Hold the plastic bottles over the shoulders in a bent-armed position.

Movement: Lower the weight toward the floor letting it come as close as possible to the forehead. Stretch in the bottom position. Return to the over-the-shoulder position and repeat.

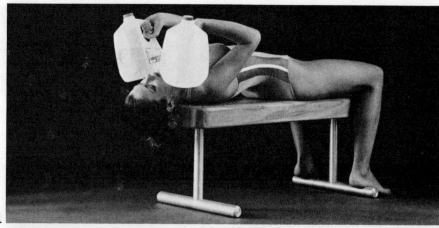

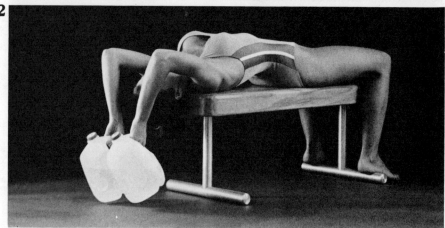

EXERCISE:
BENCH PRESS WITH PLASTIC BOTTLES

RATING: A
EQUIPMENT:
TWO WATER-FILLED PLASTIC BOTTLES

Starting Position: While seated on a narrow bench, grasp a bottle in each hand and bring them to rest on the thighs. Lie back on the bench and at the same time straighten the arms over the chest.

Movement: Lower the resistance slowly to the chest and immediately press it to the straight-armed position. Repeat until fatigued.

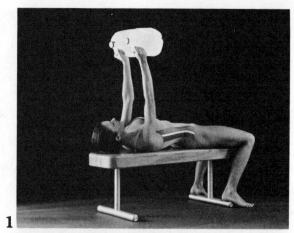

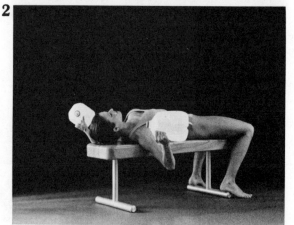

EXERCISE:
PUSHUP

RATING: B
EQUIPMENT:
NONE

Starting Position: Lie face-down on the floor with bodyweight supported on the palms of the hands and the toes. The toes should be bent and the hands should be positioned directly under the shoulders with the arms bent.

Movement: Keeping the body straight and rigid, slowly push it to arms' length. Lower and repeat.

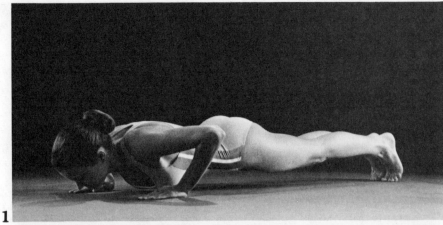

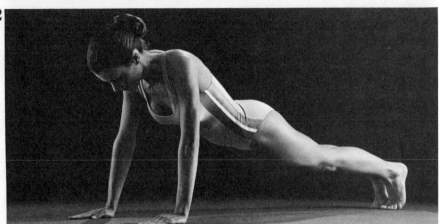

EXERCISE:
STRAIGHT-ARMED PULLOVER WITH CANS

RATING: B
EQUIPMENT:
TWO UNOPENED CANS AND BENCH

Starting Position: Lie face-up on a bench. Hold the cans over the chest in a straight-armed position.

Movement: Take a deep breath, lower the weight behind the head, and return to the over-the-chest position. It is important to keep the arms straight during the movement and to emphasize the stretching of the torso when the weight is behind the head. Repeat.

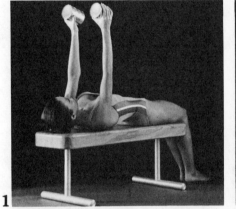
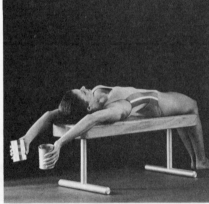
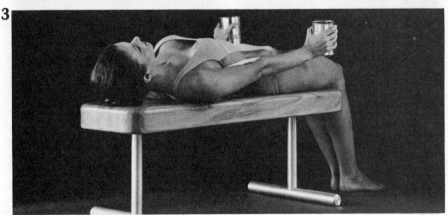

EXERCISE:
DYNAMIC CHEST
CONTRACTION

RATING: B
EQUIPMENT:
NONE

Starting Position: Match one palm with the other at a point just below and in front of the chest.

Movement: Push the two palms together as their matching position is moved back and forth across the chest.

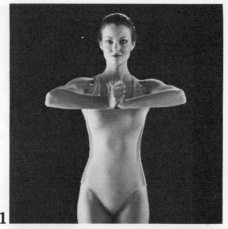

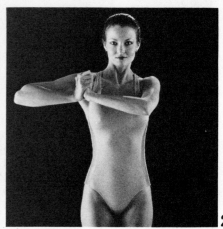

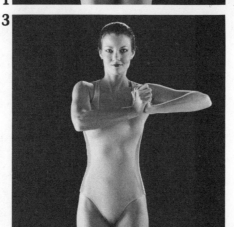

EXERCISE:
PUSHUP ON
CHAIR

RATING: B
EQUIPMENT:
CHAIR

Starting Position: Place both hands in the seat of a chair and the feet on the floor. Support the body on the palms of the hands and the toes. The arm should be bent.

Movement: Keep the body rigid and straight. Slowly push the body to arms' length, then lower. Repeat.

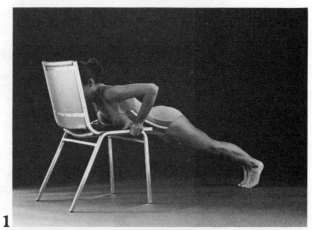

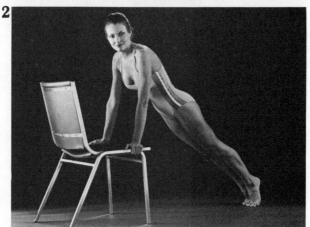

EXERCISE:
UPRIGHT ROW WITH PLASTIC BOTTLES

RATING: B

EQUIPMENT:
TWO WATER-FILLED PLASTIC BOTTLES

Starting Position: Grasp a plastic bottle in each hand. Stand erect with the arms down and straight.

Movement: Maintaining the hands close together and the palms facing the body, raise the hands to chest-height. The arms should then be bent with the elbows pointing outward. Lower and repeat.

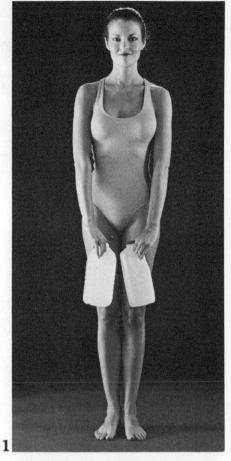

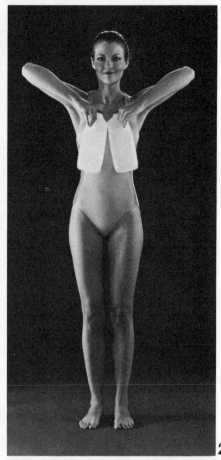

EXERCISE:
FRONT RAISE WITH CANS

RATING: B

EQUIPMENT:
TWO UNOPENED CANS

Starting Position: Grasp a can in each hand and stand erect.

Movement: Keeping the arms straight, raise the cans to shoulder height in front of the body. Pause. Slowly return to the starting position and repeat.

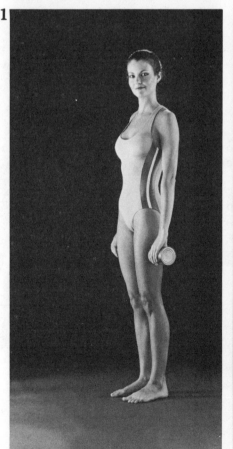

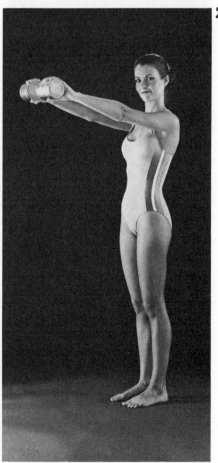

BODY SHAPING: BUST

EXERCISE:
PUSHUP ON KNEES

RATING: C
EQUIPMENT:
NONE

Starting Position: Lie face-down with the palms of the hands positioned directly under the shoulders with the arms bent.

Movement: Slowly push the body to arms' length while remaining on the knees. Lower to the floor and repeat.

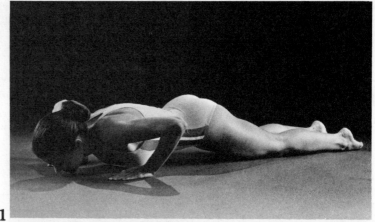

1

2

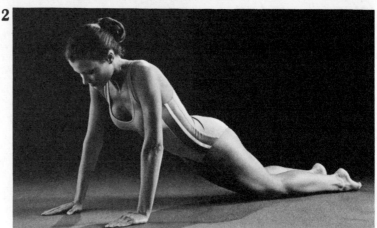

EXERCISE:
WALL PRESS

RATING: C
EQUIPMENT:
NONE

Starting Position: Lean face-first into a vertical wall at about a 45 degree angle.

Movement: With the hands positioned on the wall at shoulder height, push away until the arms are straight. Lower to meet the wall again and repeat.

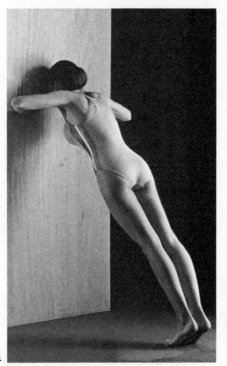

1

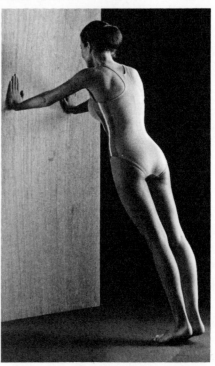

2

EXERCISE:
FRONT RAISE
WITH PLASTIC BOTTLES

RATING: C
EQUIPMENT:
TWO WATER-FILLED
PLASTIC BOTTLES

Starting Position: Grasp a bottle in each hand and stand erect.

Movement: Keeping the arms straight, raise the bottles to shoulder height in front of the body. Pause. Slowly return to the starting position and repeat.

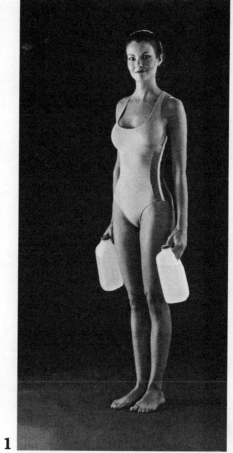

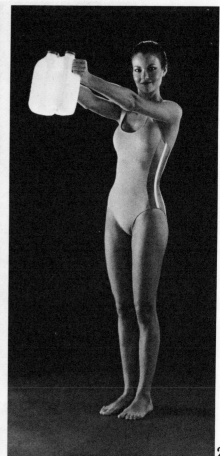

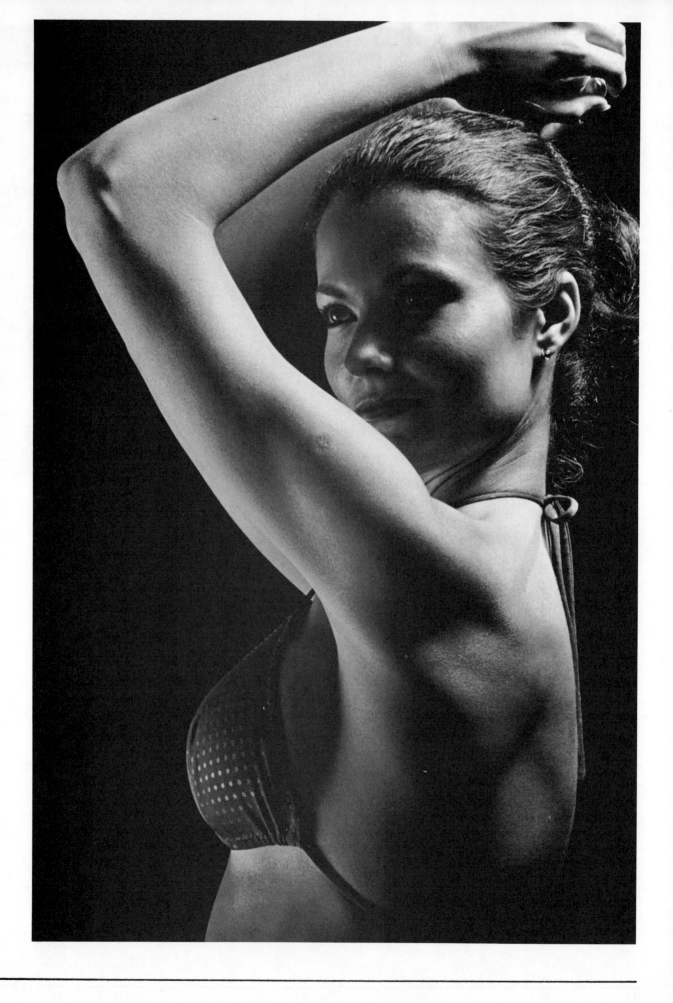

CHAPTER 9
UPPER ARMS

Most women neglect to exercise their arms. How many women regularly lift heavy loads or use their arms for strenuous exercise? And while troubled by flabby thighs and heavy hips, they rarely think about seeing that their arms are in shape. Yet upper arms are often the first part of the body to sag, no matter how fit a woman might be.

Anatomy of the Upper Arms

The upper arm is basically composed of two large muscles and thirteen smaller ones. These muscles cross the elbow joint and control its flexing and extending. Eight muscles contribute to flexion, seven to extension. The most important muscle of elbow flexion is the biceps. The most important muscle of elbow extension is the triceps.

The biceps is the prominent muscle on the front side of the upper arm. It is a two-headed muscle made up of a long and a short head. The tendons at the top end cross the shoulder joint and are attached to the scapula. At the other end, the tendons cross the elbow joint and are connected to the forearm just below the joint. The biceps cross two joints, the shoulder and the elbow. Thus, the functions of the biceps are threefold: it flexes the elbow, supinates the hand, and lifts the upper arm forward.

The triceps is on the back side of the upper arm and, as its name implies, has three separate heads: lateral, medial, and long. Like the biceps, the triceps tendons cross both the shoulder and the elbow joint. The major function of the triceps is to straighten the elbow. It also assists in bringing the upper arm down from an overhead position.

Some of the suggested exercises tone and strengthen the forearm and shoulders, as well as the upper arms. This insures symmetry among these important muscles.

BODY SHAPING

EXERCISE:
TRICEPS EXTENSION
WITH ONE CAN

RATING: A

EQUIPMENT:
ONE LARGE,
UNOPENED CAN

Starting Position: Hold a large can in the middle with both hands and raise it overhead. Keep the elbow by the ears.

Movement: Slowly bend and straighten the arms. Do not move the elbows. Repeat.

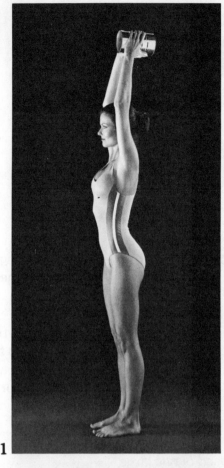

1

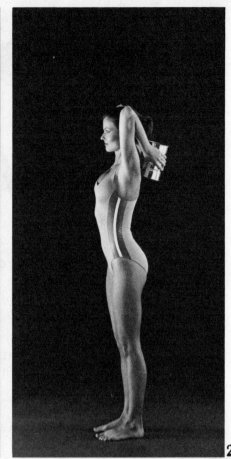

2

EXERCISE:
TRICEPS EXTENSION
WITH CANS

RATING: A

EQUIPMENT:
TWO UNOPENED CANS

Starting Position: Grasp a can in each hand and raise it overhead. Keep the elbows by the ears.

Movement: Slowly bend and straighten the arms. Do not move the elbows. Repeat.

1

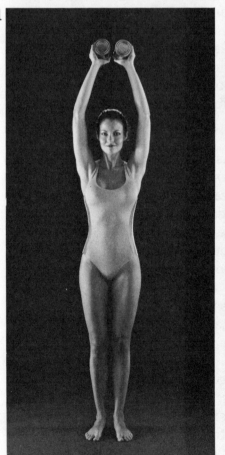

2

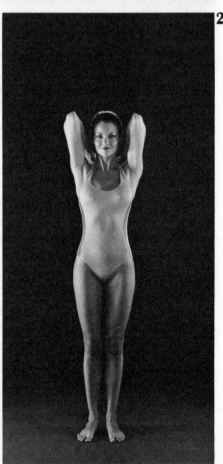

EXERCISE:
BICEPS CURL
WITH CANS

RATING: A
EQUIPMENT:
TWO CANS

Starting Position: Grasp a can in each hand with the palms up. Stand erect.

Movement: While keeping the body straight, smoothly curl the cans. Slowly lower and repeat.

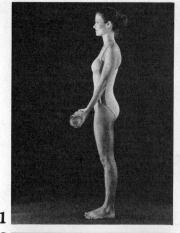

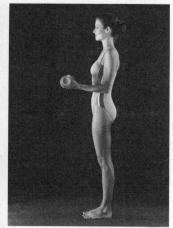

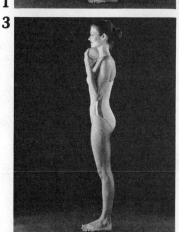

EXERCISE:
SEATED ONE-ARMED
CURL WITH CAN

RATING: A
EQUIPMENT:
UNOPENED CAN
AND CHAIR

Starting Position: Sit on the edge of a chair. Grasp an unopened can in the right hand. Lean forward and immobilize the right elbow by planting it on the inside surface of the right thigh.

Movement: Starting with the arm hanging, curl the can to the shoulder. Pause. Slowly lower and repeat. When fatigued, switch to the left arm.

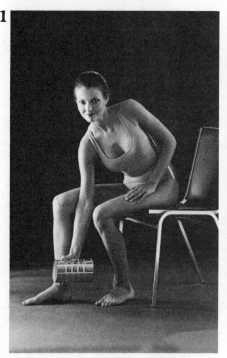

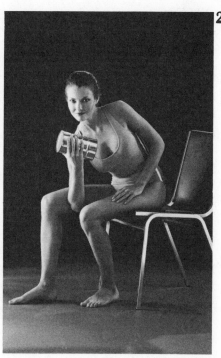

95

EXERCISE:
CHINUP

RATING: A
EQUIPMENT:
HORIZONTAL BAR

Starting Position: Grasp the horizontal bar with the palms facing the body. Hang.

Movement: Pull the body upward so that the chin is over the bar. Pause. Slowly lower the body to the starting position and repeat.

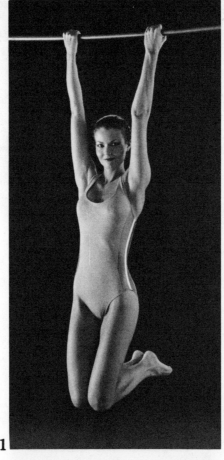

1

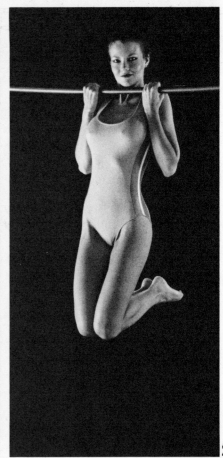

2

EXERCISE:
NEGATIVE CHINUP

RATING: A
EQUIPMENT:
HORIZONTAL BAR
AND CHAIR

Starting Position: Place a chair under the horizontal bar. Grasp the bar with palms facing the body. Using the chair, climb to the top position with the chin over the bar. Release the legs by bending the knees.

Movement: Slowly lower the body to the hanging position by unbending the arms. Climb back to the top position and repeat.

1

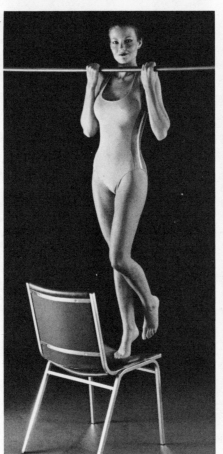

2

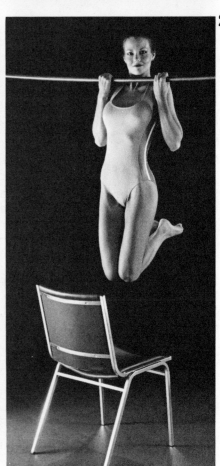

EXERCISE:
STANDING CHAIR DIP

RATING: A

EQUIPMENT:
TWO CHAIRS

Starting Position: Face two chairs away from each other. Stand between them. Support the body on straightened arms against the backs of the chairs. Bend the legs at the knees.

Movement: Slowly lower the body by bending the arms. Stretch in the lowest position and smoothly return to the top. Repeat.

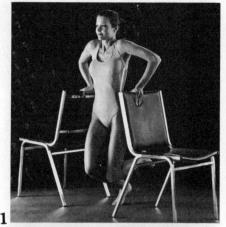

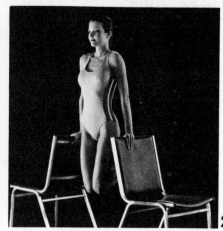

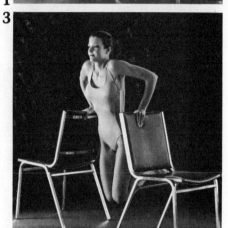

EXERCISE:
OVERHEAD PRESS WITH CANS

RATING: B

EQUIPMENT:
TWO UNOPENED CANS

Starting Position: Grasp a can in each hand and bring them to the shoulders.

Movement: Press the cans overhead and lower slowly back to the shoulders. Repeat.

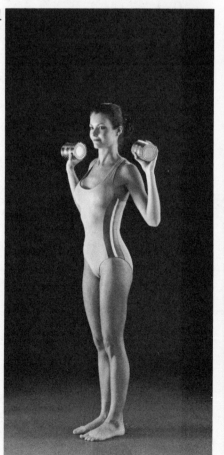

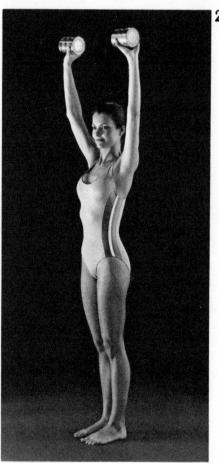

BODY SHAPING: UPPER ARMS

EXERCISE:
REVERSE CURL WITH CANS

RATING: B
EQUIPMENT:
TWO UNOPENED CANS

Starting Position: Grasp a can in each hand.

Movement: Keeping the palms down and elbows immobilized in the ribs, bend the arms. Slowly lower and repeat.

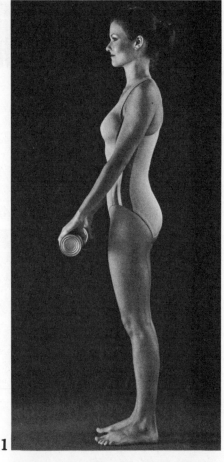 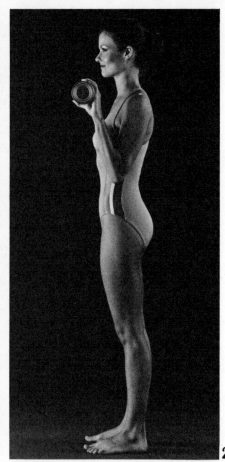

EXERCISE:
TRICEPS EXTENSION WITH TOWEL

RATING: B
EQUIPMENT:
TOWEL

Starting Position: Grasp a towel with both hands in such a manner that the towel travels behind the head. One arm is fully bent as the other is fully straightened. The towel should not touch the back of the head.

Movement: Alternately straighten and bend both arms. The resistance of one arm will be provided by the force of the other. Repeat until fatigued.

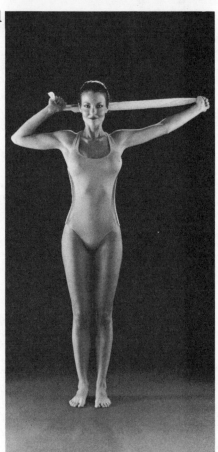 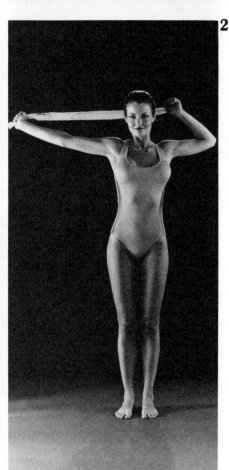

EXERCISE:
LYING CHINUP

RATING: B

EQUIPMENT:
BROOM HANDLE AND
TWO CHAIRS

Starting Position: Span an approximate two-foot distance between two chairs with a broom handle across the backs. Position the upper body under the broom handle. Grasp the handle with the palms facing the body.

Movement: Pull the chest to the broom handle. Pause and then lower slowly. Keep the body straight. Only the heels should touch the floor. If too difficult, allow the body to bend slightly as it is lifted, then keep it straight and rigid as it is lowered. Repeat.

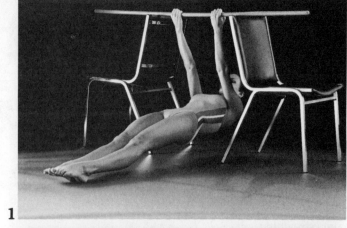

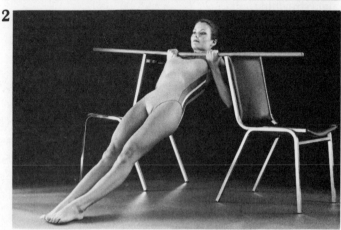

EXERCISE:
PARTNER-ASSISTED
TRICEPS EXTENSION

RATING: B

EQUIPMENT:
TOWEL, CHAIR
AND PARTNER

Starting Position: Sit in a chair and have a partner kneeling behind. The elbows should be by the ears with one end of a towel held firmly in both hands. The partner grasps the other end of the towel and takes up the slack.

Movement: Smoothly straighten and bend the arms as the partner provides the resistance by pulling on the towel. Repeat until fatigued.

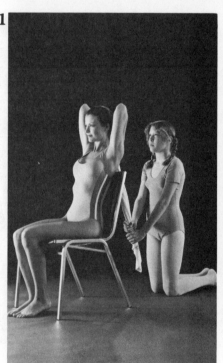

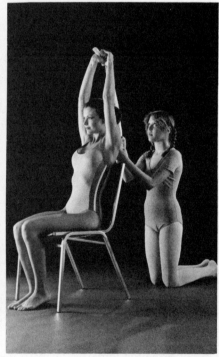

BODY SHAPING: UPPER ARMS

EXERCISE:
CHAIR-SEAT DIP

RATING: B
EQUIPMENT:
CHAIR

Starting Position: Place the palms on the front edge of a chair. The heels of the feet should rest on the floor in front. Attempt to sit on the floor in front of the chair.

Movement: Alternately straighten and bend the arms, lifting and lowering the body. Repeat until fatigued.

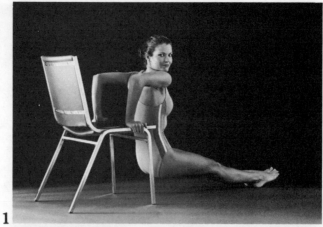

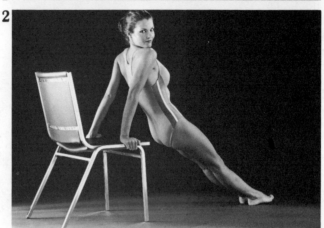

EXERCISE:
WRIST CURL WITH PLASTIC BOTTLE

RATING: C
EQUIPMENT:
BROOM HANDLE AND PLASTIC BOTTLE

Starting Position: Slide bottle to middle of broom handle. Grasp the handle on both sides of the bottle with a palms-up grip. Rest the forearms on the thighs and the backs of the hands against the knees and be seated. Lean forward until the angle between the upper arms and forearms is less then 90 degrees.

Movement: Smoothly curl the hands and contract the forearm muscles. Pause and slowly lower the resistance. Do not allow the forearms or torso to move. Do not extend the fingers. Keep the handle in the palms of the hands. Repeat.

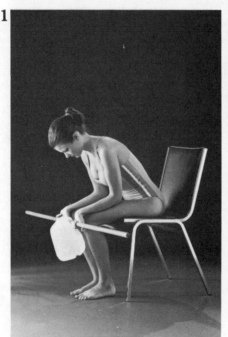

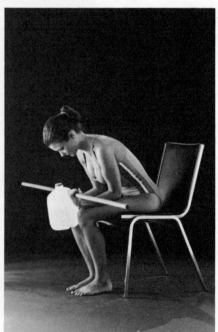

EXERCISE:
REVERSE WRIST CURL WITH PLASTIC BOTTLE

RATING: C
EQUIPMENT:
BROOM HANDLE AND PLASTIC BOTTLE

Starting Position: Slide bottle to middle of broom handle. Grasp the handle with a palms-down grip. Rest the forearms on the thighs and wrists of the hands against the knees and be seated. Lean forward until the angle between the upper arms and forearms is less than 90 degrees.

Movement: Smoothly move the hands upward. Pause. Slowly lower to the starting position and repeat.

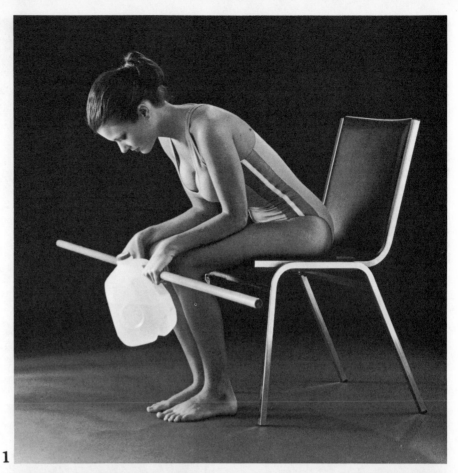

1

2

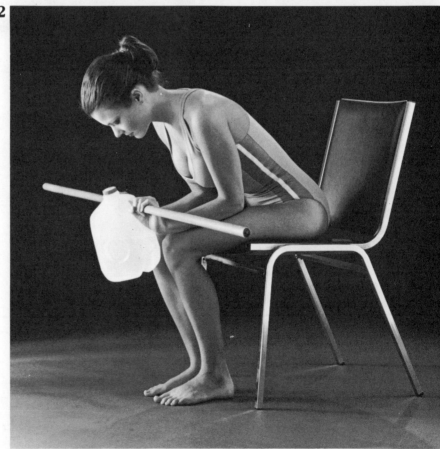

EXERCISE:
NEWSPAPER WADDING

RATING: C
EQUIPMENT:
SHEETS OF NEWSPAPER

Starting Position: Stand erect. Grasp the middle of a full-size sheet of newspaper.

Movement: Wad the newspaper as quickly as possible with the right hand only. Repeat several times. Now try the left hand.

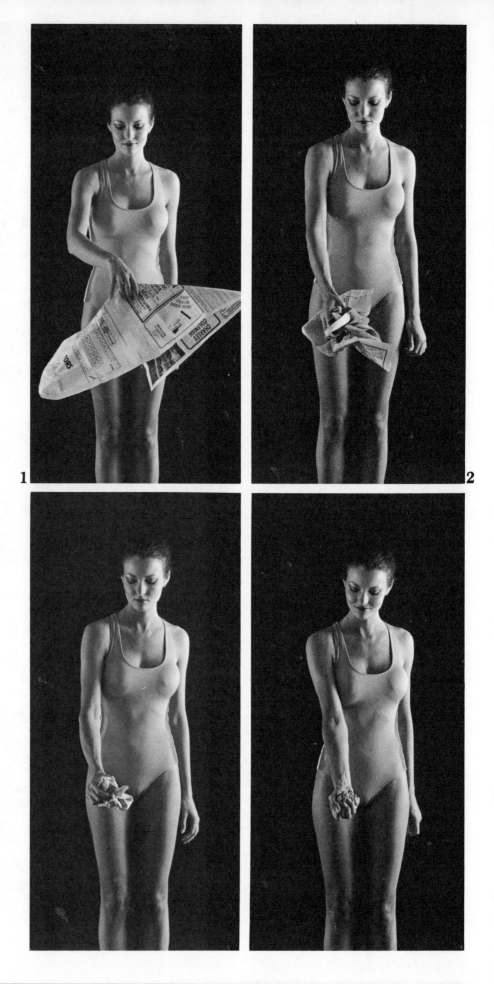

EXERCISE:
FINGER CURL WITH
PLASTIC BOTTLE

RATING: C
EQUIPMENT:
BROOM HANDLE AND
PLASTIC BOTTLE

Starting Position: Slide bottle to middle of broom handle. Grasp the handle on both sides of the bottle with a palms-up grip. Rest the forearms on the thighs and backs of the hands against the knees and be seated. Lean forward until the angle between the upper arms and forearms is less than 90 degrees.

Movement: Instead of moving the hands and flexing the wrists, simply extend the fingers. Curl the fingers and repeat.

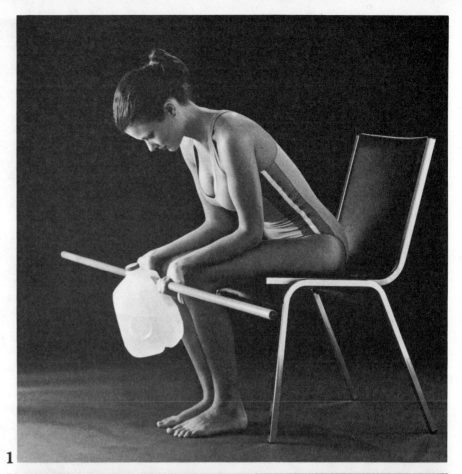

1

2

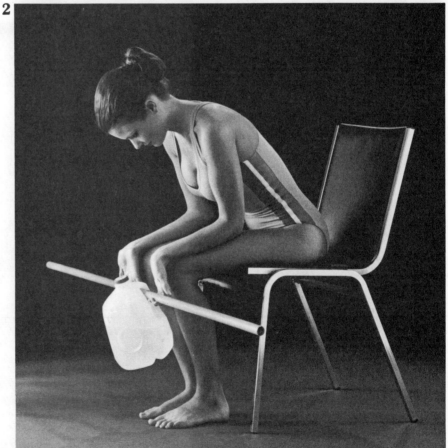

BODY SHAPING: UPPER ARMS

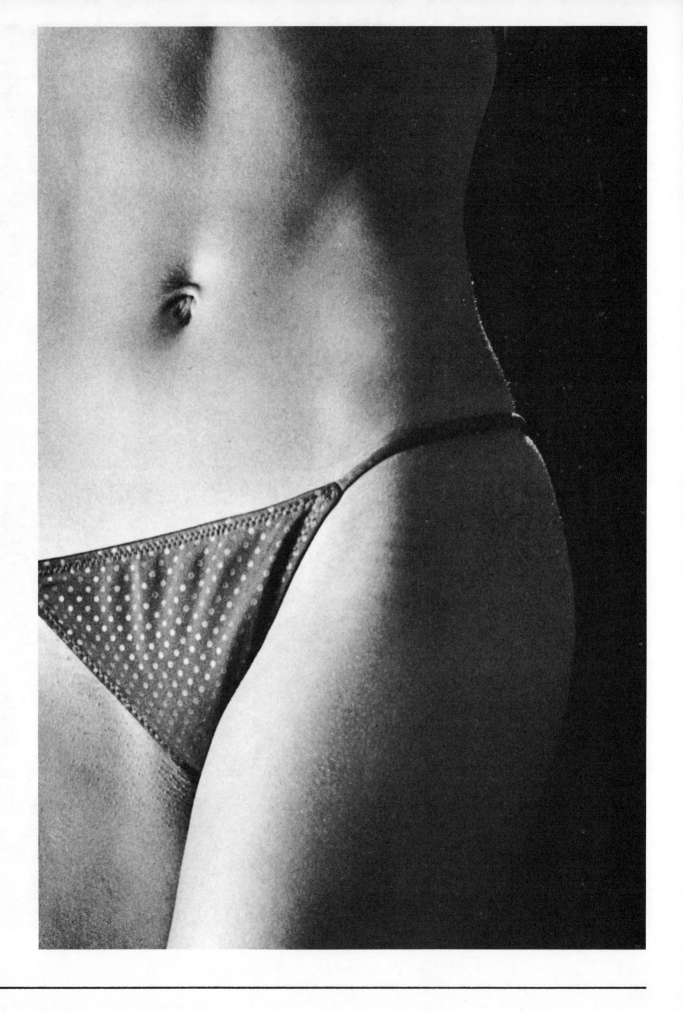

CHAPTER 10
WAIST

Nothing can do more to upset the lines of an otherwise attractive figure than a sloppy waistline. The renowned pot belly is not only unattractive and aging in appearance, but it is often a prelude to future illness.

Few features stand out in a bathing suit as much as a slim, trim waistline. In clothes a slender waist can make a woman's positive traits more alluring and the negative ones less noticeable.

Witness the appeal of the glamour crowd in show business. The most popular male and female stars all have firm, flat middles: Farrah Fawcett, Burt Reynolds, Cheryl Tiegs, Clint Eastwood, Robert Redford, Kate Jackson, O.J. Simpson, Olivia Newton-John, John Travolta, Jaclyn Smith, Mick Jagger, Lynda Carter, Tom Jones, Cheryl Ladd and Bo Derek.

A trim waist makes the bustline look fuller and gives the woman a healthy, athletic appearance. If women want to increase their sex appeal, reducing that fatty tissue around the waistline and strengthening the muscles of the midsection will increase their appeal to the opposite sex.

Anatomy of the Waist

The appearance and strength of the waist is primarily determined by three muscles: rectus abdominis, external oblique, and internal oblique. The rectus abdominis is attached to the fifth, sixth, and seventh ribs, extends across the front of the abdominal wall, and joins the pubis bone. The external and internal obliques cover both sides of the abdomen. They are attached to the lower ribs and extend to the crest of the hip bone. The primary functions of the abdominal group are to flex the spinal column forward and side to side.

The belief that situps and leg raises are abdominal exercises is a misconception. These movements work the hip flexors. The hip flexors connect the upper femur bones of the thighs to the lower lumbar region of the spine. When these muscles contract they pull the upper body to a sitting position, or pull the thighs up toward the chest as in a leg raise. The abdominals are only mildly involved in a traditional situp or leg raise.

The function of the rectus abdominis muscle is to shorten the distance between the sternum and hips. To accomplish this lie flat on the back. Roll the shoulders and head forward. At the same time raise the hips upward and back toward the chest. This contraction is the primary function of the abdominals.

To isolate the hip flexors so that they are not inadvertently used, spread the knees and move the heels up toward the buttocks. While in this position place the hands behind the neck and perform quarter situps. Do not allow the feet and legs to be held down by a partner, strap, or other apparatus.

Another common misconception is that the midsection will be reduced if subjected to more repetitions than other body parts. Many people perform situps and leg raises by the hundreds in the mistaken belief that they will assist in burning fat and defining the waistline. Exercise for the midsection has no effect on fat loss in the waist. It cannot be emphasized too often that spot reduction is not possible. The abdominals should be treated as any other muscle group. One set of 8-12 repetitions should be performed each workout. When 12 or more repetitions can be performed correctly, resistance should be added.

BODY SHAPING

EXERCISE:
TRUNK CURL

RATING: A
EQUIPMENT:
NONE

Starting Position: Lie face-up on the floor with the hands behind the head. Bring the heels close to the buttocks and spread the knees.

Movement: Try to curl the trunk to a sitting position. Only one-third of a standard situp can be performed in this fashion. Pause in the contracted position. Slowly lower the trunk to the floor and repeat.

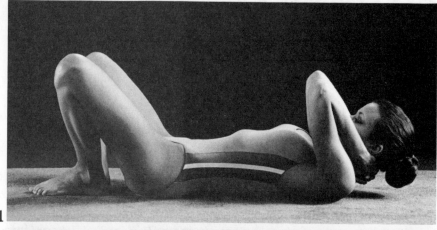

1

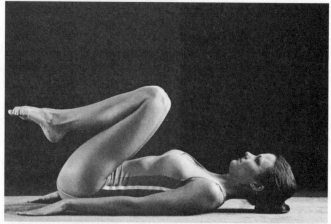

2

EXERCISE:
REVERSE
TRUNK CURL

RATING: A
EQUIPMENT:
NONE

Starting Position: Lie face-up on the floor with the hands on either side of the buttocks. Bring the thighs on the chest so the knees and hips are in a flexed position.

Movement: Curl the pelvic area toward the chin by lifting the buttocks and lower back. Pause. Slowly lower the buttocks and repeat.

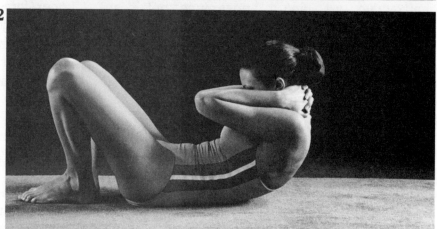

1

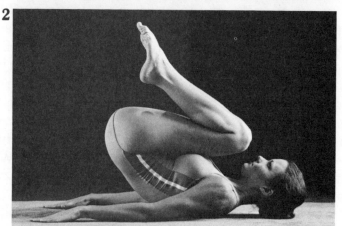

2

EXERCISE:
NEGATIVE
TRUNK CURL

RATING: A
EQUIPMENT:
CHAIR

Starting Position: Lie face-up on the floor with the lower legs in the seat of the chair. In this position, the thighs should be vertical.

Movement: Use the elbows and hands, pushing first on the floor, then pulling on the legs of the chair. Raise the head and shoulders toward the knees as far as possible. Without moving the head and shoulders, release the hands and interlace them behind the head. Lower the shoulders to the floor very slowly and repeat.

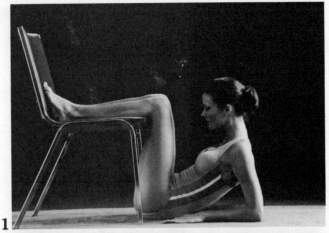

1

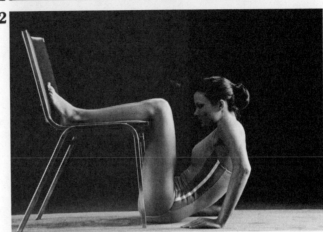

2

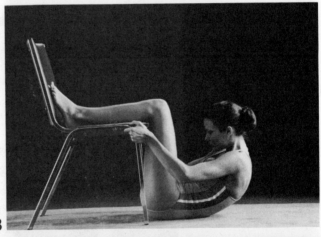

3

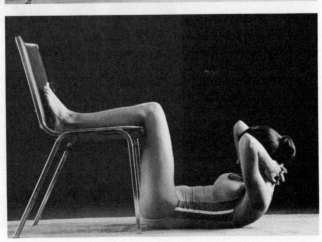

4

107

BODY SHAPING: WAIST

EXERCISE:
SIDE BEND WITH PLASTIC BOTTLE

RATING: A
EQUIPMENT:
WATER-FILLED PLASTIC BOTTLE

Starting Position: Grasp bottle in right hand and stand erect. Place left hand on top of head.

Movement: Bend to the right side as far as possible. Return to the standing position and repeat. Change hands and work left side.

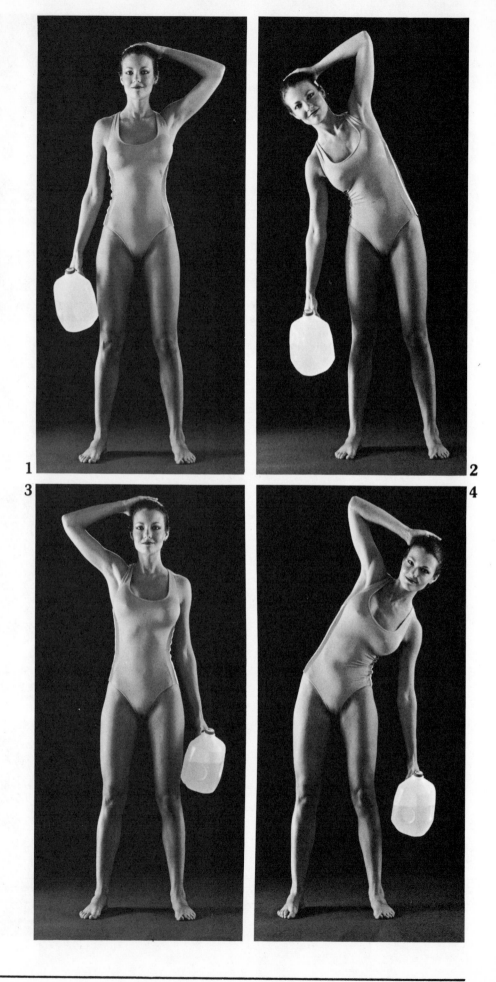

EXERCISE:
V-UP

RATING: B
EQUIPMENT:
NONE

Starting Position: Lie face-up on the floor with the hands at the side of the buttocks and the legs straight.

Movement: Keeping the legs and arms straight, slowly try to touch the hands to the feet. The body will be supported on the buttocks. Pause. Slowly lower and repeat.

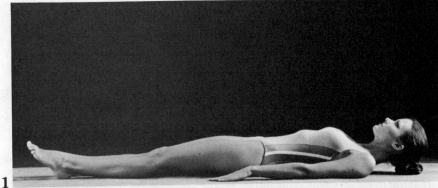

1

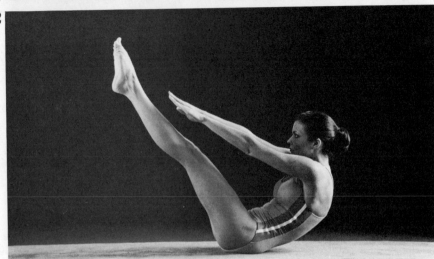

2

EXERCISE:
SIDE
TRUNK CURL

RATING: B
EQUIPMENT:
BENCH AND PARTNER

Starting Position: Lie on a bench facing sideways. The body should be supported at one side of the buttocks as a partner holds the feet down. The bench edge should coincide with the waist.

Movement: Laterally curl the upper body as high as possible. Pause, then lower it **slowly** and repeat. Switch sides.

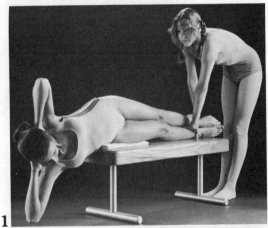

1

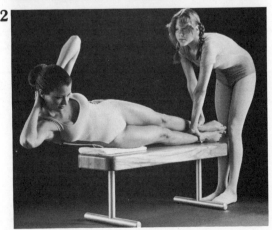

2

BODY SHAPING: WAIST

EXERCISE:
TWISTING TRUNK CURL

RATING: B
EQUIPMENT: NONE

Starting Position: Lie face-up on the floor with the hands behind the head. Bring the heels up close to the buttocks and spread the knees. Curl the trunk to the contracted position.

Movement: In the contracted position, twist back and forth at the waist until fatigued.

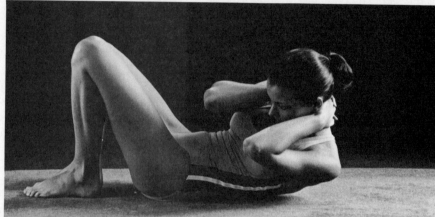

1

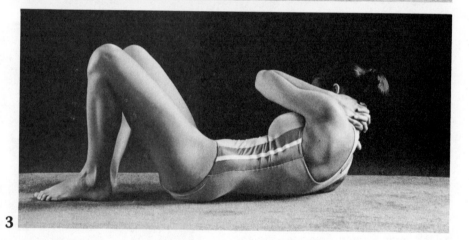

2

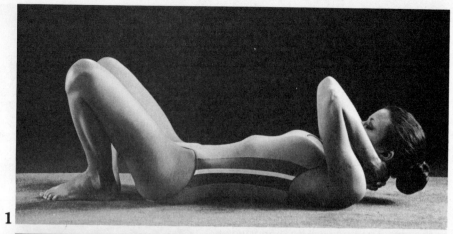

3

EXERCISE:
SIDE BEND WITH TOWEL

RATING: B
EQUIPMENT:
TOWEL

Starting Position: Grasp towel at each end and raise overhead. Stand with the feet shoulder-width apart.

Movement: Bend to the right side as far as possible. Return to the vertical position and bend to the left side as far as possible. Return to the vertical position and repeat.

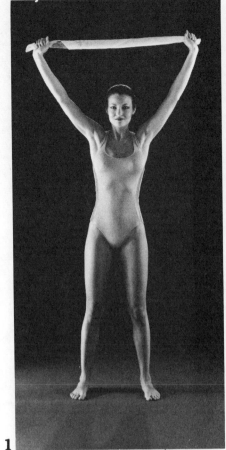

1

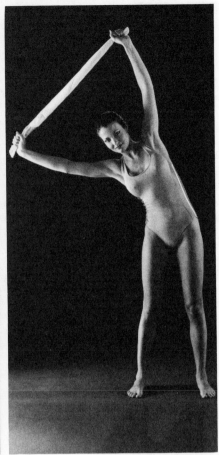

2

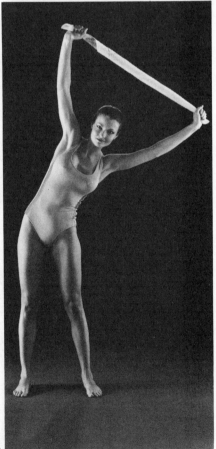

3

BODY SHAPING: WAIST

EXERCISE:
TWISTING REVERSE
TRUNK CURL

RATING: B
EQUIPMENT:
NONE

Starting Position: Lie face-up on the floor with the hands on either side of the buttocks. Bring the thighs on the chest so that the knees and hips are in a flexed position. Curl the pelvic area toward the chin by lifting the buttocks and lower back.

Movement: Maintaining everything else, twist back and forth at the waist. Repeat until fatigued.

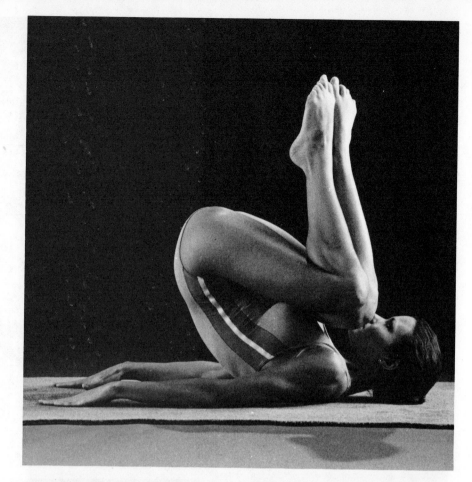

EXERCISE:
SIDE BEND

RATING: B
EQUIPMENT:
NONE

Starting Position: Stand with the feet slightly apart and link the hands on the head.

Movement: Bend to the right side as far as possible. Return to the vertical position and bend to the left side as far as possible. Return to the vertical position and repeat. Additional resistance can be held in the hands overhead.

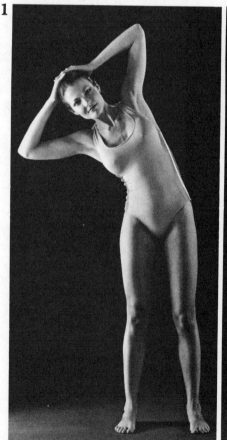
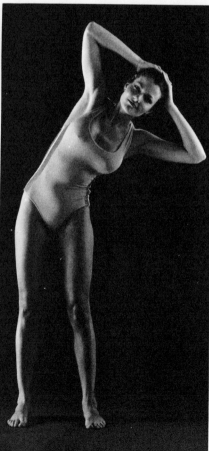

EXERCISE:
LEG RAISE
IN CHAIR

RATING: C
EQUIPMENT:
CHAIR

Starting Position: Sit erect in a chair with the feet on the floor directly in front. Grasp the sides of the seat for stabilization.

Movement: Lift the knees to the chest and pause. Lower and repeat.

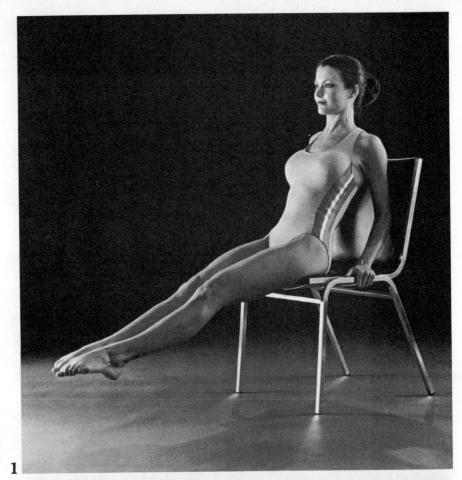

1

2

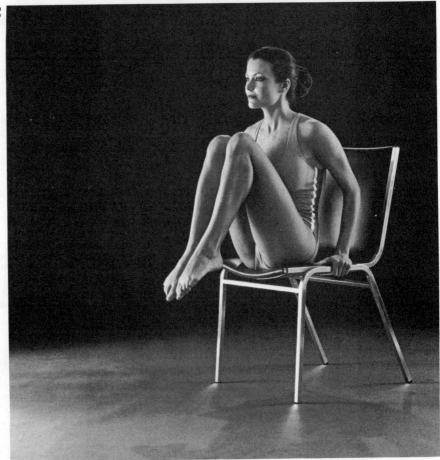

BODY SHAPING: WAIST

EXERCISE:
CHAIR TWIST

RATING: C
EQUIPMENT:
CHAIR

Starting Position: Sit in a chair. The left hand holds the right upper edge of the chair. The right hand holds the other edge. Both elbows should be down.

Movement: Press with the left hand, pull with the right, and gently twist the torso to the left. Hold the stretched position for about 15 seconds. Change positions to stretch the right side.

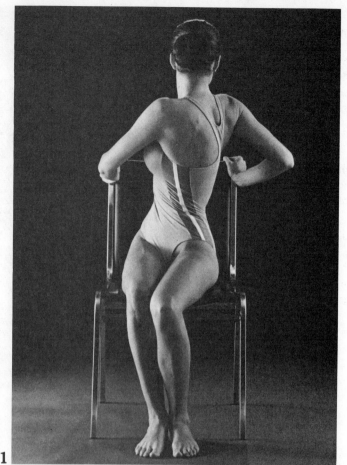

1

2

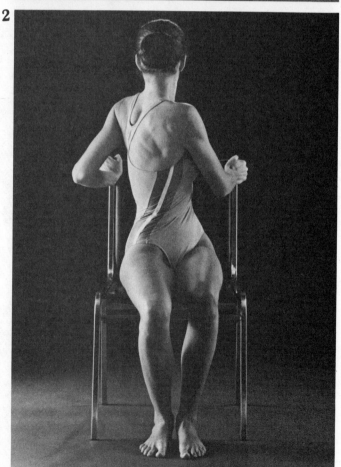

EXERCISE:
LEG CROSSOVER TRUNK ROLL

RATING: C
EQUIPMENT: NONE

Starting Position: Lie face-up on the floor with the hands on either side of the shoulders. Legs should be straight.

Movement: Cross one leg over the other causing the hip to rotate and the waist to twist. Keep the shoulders and arms on the floor. Return to starting position and repeat until fatigued. Then perform with the other leg.

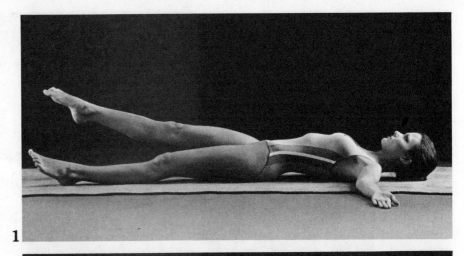

1

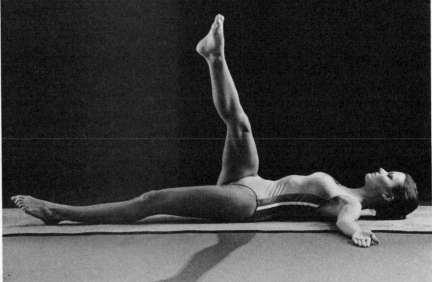

2

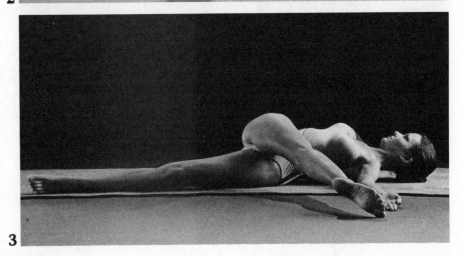

3

BODY SHAPING: WAIST

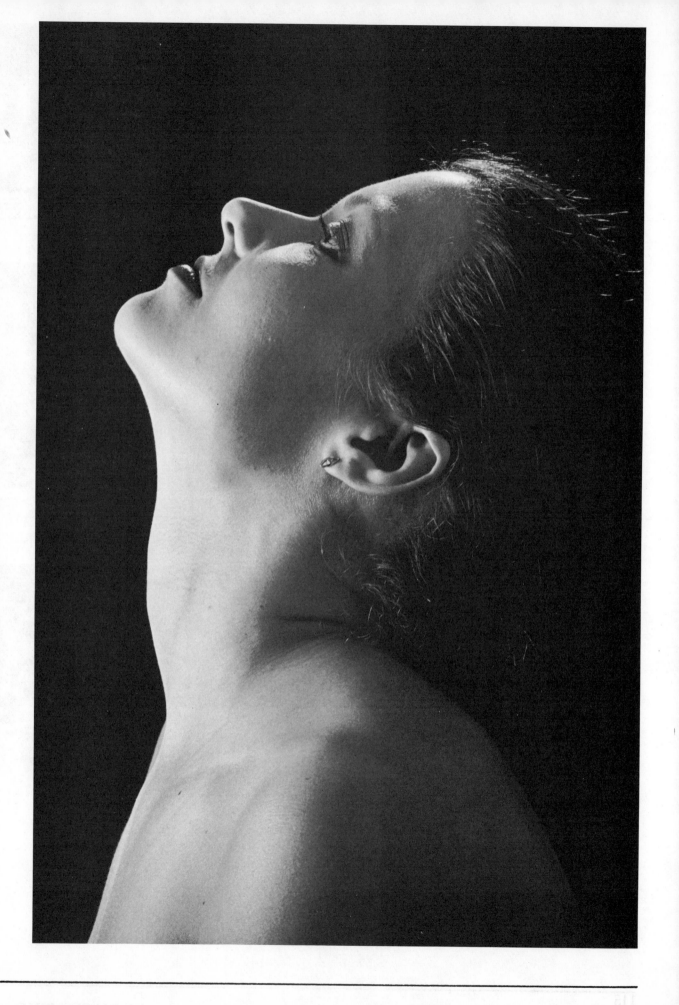

CHAPTER 11
FACE & NECK

The face and neck are the most visible parts of a woman's body. They present an open testimony to her emotions, moods, state of health, and frequently her age.

Most women tend to think that wrinkles alone signify an aging face. But perhaps more dramatic and noticeable evidence of aging is a loose, sagging face. Shrinking around the eyes, slack cheeks, drooping corners of the mouth, flabby skin beneath the jaw, and a furrowed upper lip can be very unattractive. These unpleasant characteristics are primarily the result of atrophied muscles and facial flesh.

Both wrinkles and sagging skin are inevitable to all adults. They are bound to appear sooner or later depending on such things as skin type, genetic tendencies, general state of health, and exposure to the elements. Even though there is not much a woman can do to erase wrinkles, the slack muscles of the face can be strengthened, like sagging muscles anywhere in the body, with proper exercise.

Next to the facial muscles, the most neglected muscles of the feminine figure are those of the neck. A scrawny neck stands out conspicuously even in the best built woman. A shapely and strong neck is not only an addition to personal appearance, it is a valuable safeguard against injury. Whiplash and other neck injuries happen to thousands of women every week as a result of minor accidents. Many of these injuries would not have happened if the victim had had a stronger neck. Even in simple weekend activities, there are many cases of preventable stiff necks.

Anatomy of the Face and Neck

It is a surprise for many women to learn that the face is crisscrossed with at least 16 muscles. These muscles are not tiny and insignificant, but are large and powerful. Only the temples, skull, and small spots on the chin and the center of the nose are totally without muscles.

Some of the facial muscles, such as those used to smile and chew, get regular exercise. But the majority of the muscles in the face never move of their own accord. They are merely pulled along when habitual facial expressions are made. A woman's eyes, for example, are ringed by powerful muscles. When she opens and closes them, however, she uses only the muscles in the upper lids. The muscles in the lower lids merely get pulled along. These inactive facial muscles can be compared to the muscles in the average person's toes. The toes usually get a free ride from the muscles of the hips, thighs, and calves and do little work of their own. It is no wonder that most Americans have problems with their feet.

Muscles are responsible for keeping the face smooth. If an individual allows the facial muscles to atrophy as she ages, the spaces between the muscle and the skin will increase, creating sags. If a woman learns to exercise the atrophying muscles of the face, they will increase in strength and shape. When the sagging skin is drawn taut again, the face will become smoother and more attractive.

The lack of strength and muscle tone in the face also carries over to the neck. When humans assumed the upright position, the huge muscles at the nape of the neck wasted away. Now the average woman balances her head, weighing about 12 pounds, upon seven small cervical vertebrae. The only restraining elements that oppose sudden movements of the neck are the strength and integrity of the cervical vertebrae, the spinal ligaments, and the neck muscles. It is essential, therfore, to strengthen and develop this protective musculature.

At least 15 muscles make up the majority of the neck's musculature. These muscles are capable of producing movement in seven different directions:
(1) Elevating the shoulders
(2) Bending the head down toward the chest
(3) Drawing the head backward
(4) Bending the head down toward the right shoulder
(5) Bending the head down toward the left shoulder
(6) Twisting the head to look over the right shoulder
(7) Twisting the head to look over the left shoulder

When full-range exercise is provided for these seven functions, the response of the neck ·muscles is immediate. Both the neck and the face respond quickly to exercise because these muscles are exposed to so little hard work.

EXERCISE:
POINT THE FACE

RATING: A
EQUIPMENT:
NONE

Starting Position: Stand in front of a mirror.

Movement: Try to make the eyes, nose, chin, and cheeks squeeze to a point in the center of the face. Be sure to pucker the lips, flatten the chin, and wrinkle the bridge of the nose. Squeeze, pause, release, and repeat.

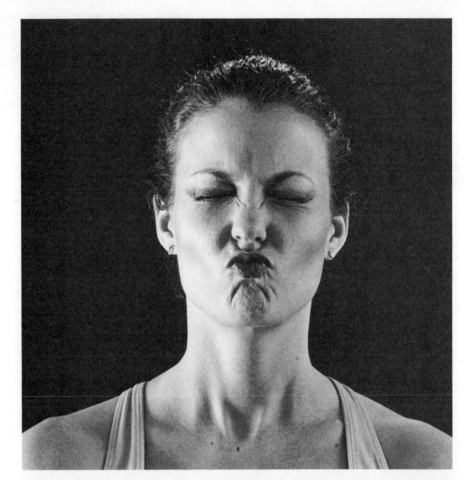

EXERCISE:
NOSE RAISE

RATING: A
EQUIPMENT:
NONE

Starting Position: Stand and look into a mirror.

Movement: Raise the upper lip. Feel the tightness develop around the nose. Do not use the cheeks. Lower the upper lip so as to pull the nose downward. Do not part the lips, or extend the upper lip over the lower. Repeat for one minute.

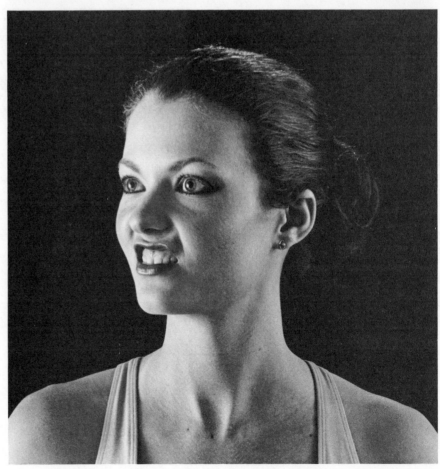

BODY SHAPING: FACE AND NECK

EXERCISE:
FOREHEAD SLIDE

RATING: A
EQUIPMENT:
NONE

Starting Position: Apply the index fingers directly under the eyebrows. The fingertips should rest at the roof of the nose.

Movement: Press the forehead down as the fingers remain in place. Keep the neck aligned with the spine. Make the muscles of the forehead do the work. Repeat for one minute.

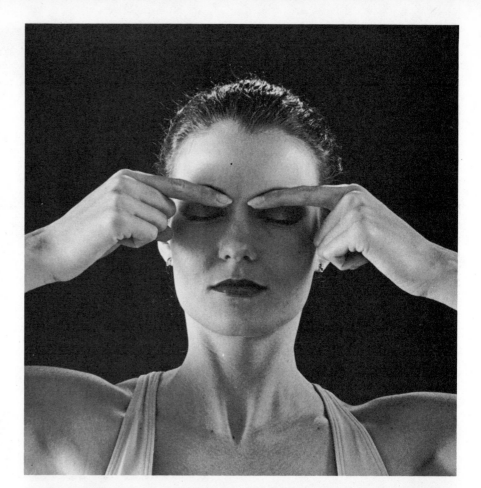

EXERCISE:
LOWER LID CLOSE

RATING A
EQUIPMENT:
NONE

Starting Position: Look straight ahead and maintain open eyes. Do not force them open or use any but the eye muscles.

Movement: Slowly move the lower eyelid up and down. This may require concentration and practice. Try not to involve the cheeks and eyebrows. Do not close the eyes as in squinting, but imagine trying to close the eyes with the lower lid as opposed to the upper. Repeat for one minute.

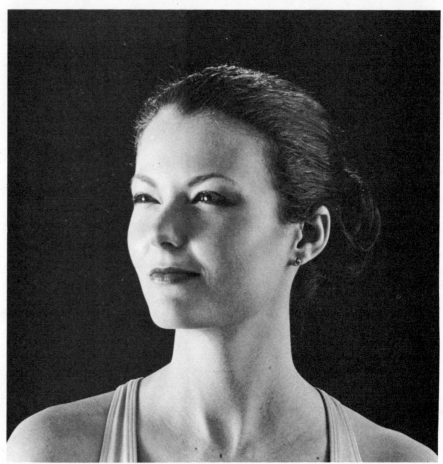

EXERCISE:
JAW PULL

RATING: A
EQUIPMENT:
NONE

Starting Position: Drop the lower jaw by relaxing it. Hook three fingers behind and upon the lower teeth.

Movement: Pull the lower jaw down further. Close the jaw slowly, without clamping fingers and then stretch against the resistance provided by the fingers and hand. Repeat.
Hint: Do not stick out the neck; keep it in line with the spine. Extension of the neck prevents effective isolation in the exercise.

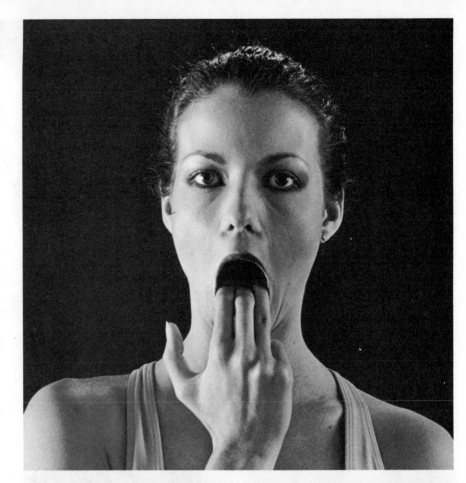

EXERCISE:
FRONT NECK
FLEXION AGAINST
HAND RESISTANCE

RATING: A
EQUIPMENT:
NONE

Starting Position: Interlace the fingers and place them on the forehead.

Movement: Move the head forward against the resistance of the hands and arms. When the chin is on the chest, use the arms to push the head backward. Continue this forward and backward motion until fatigued.

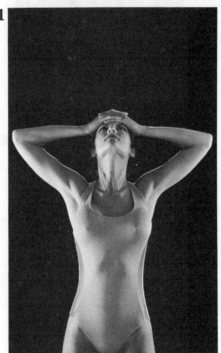

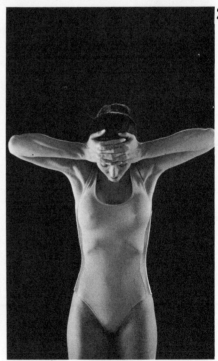

BODY SHAPING: FACE AND NECK

EXERCISE:
WEB NECK

RATING: A
EQUIPMENT:
NONE

Starting Position: Stand and look into the mirror.

Movement: Pull the corners of the mouth down as the chin points upward. Release. Try one corner only then the other for variation. This should bring out the sheet of superficial muscle overlaying the front of the neck. Repeat for one minute.

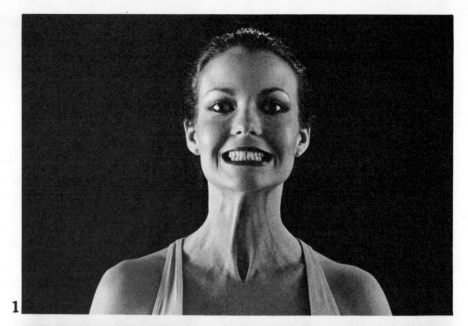

1

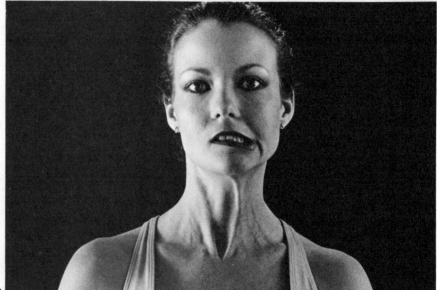

2

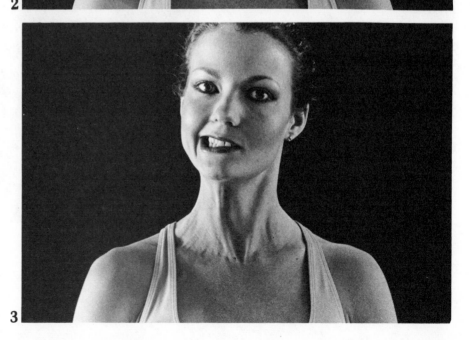

3

EXERCISE:
REAR NECK EXTENSION AGAINST HAND RESISTANCE

RATING: A
EQUIPMENT: NONE

Starting Position: Interlace the fingers and place them on the back of the head. Chin should be on chest.

Movement: Push head back and resist the movement by pulling with the arms. Then pull forward with the arms and resist with neck muscles. Repeat.

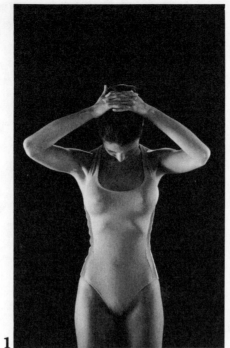

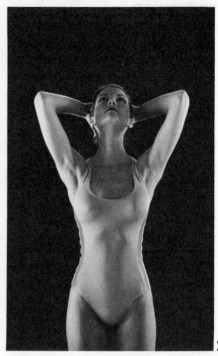

EXERCISE:
SIDE NECK FLEXION AGAINST HAND RESISTANCE

RATING: A
EQUIPMENT: NONE

Starting Position: With the head resting on the right shoulder, place the right hand just above the right ear.

Movement: Push the head to the left as far as it will go while resisting with the neck. Then use the neck to push the arm back to the starting position while resisting with the arm. After the right side of the neck is fatigued, reverse the procedure and work the left side of the neck against the left arm.

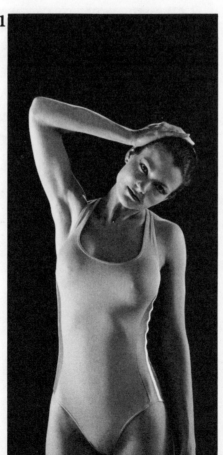

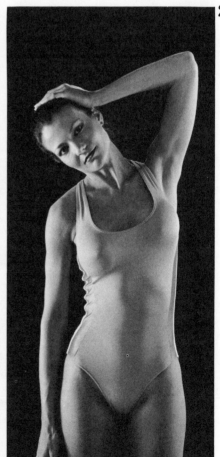

EXERCISE:
SHOULDER SHRUG WITH PLASTIC BOTTLES

RATING: A
EQUIPMENT:
TWO WATER-FILLED PLASTIC BOTTLES

Starting Position: Grasp the plastic bottles and stand.

Movement: Keeping the arms straight, smoothly shrug the shoulders as high as possible. Pause in the top position. Slowly lower and repeat.

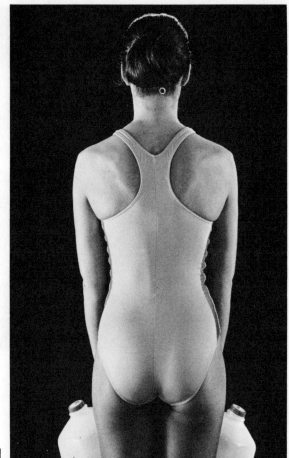

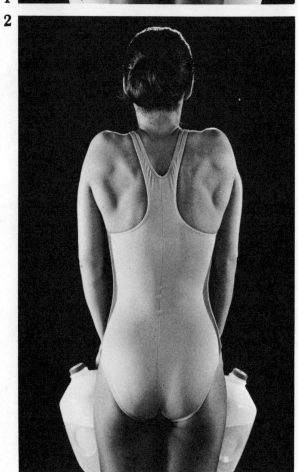

EXERCISE:
NECK ROTATION
AGAINST HAND
RESISTANCE

RATING: B
EQUIPMENT:
NONE

Starting Position: Place each hand on the corresponding side of the face.

Movement: Turn the head against the force of the hands. Perform both directions for one minute.

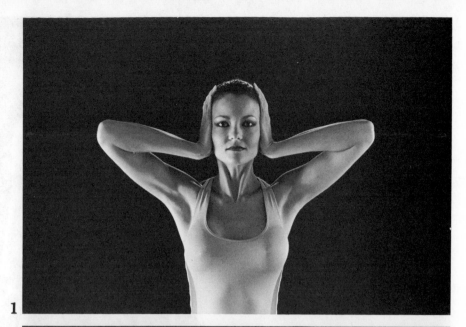

1

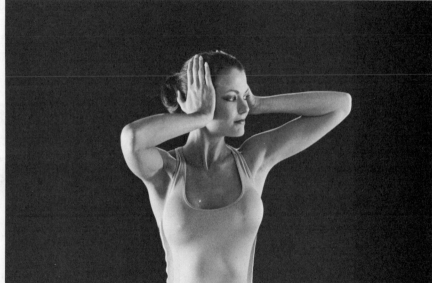

2

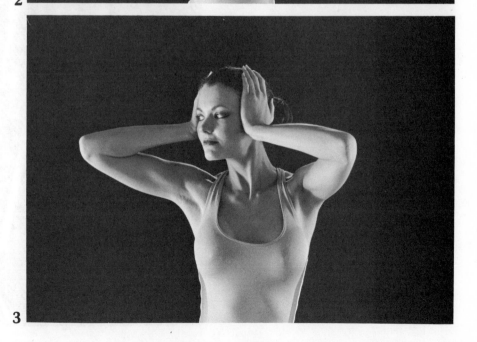

3

EXERCISE:
TORSO SHRUG

RATING: B
EQUIPMENT:
TWO CHAIRS

Starting Position: Face two chairs away from each other. Stand between them with their backs directly under the shoulders. Support the body with the straightened arms, palms on the backs of the chairs.

Movement: Keep the arms locked as the shoulders alone raise the body up and down.

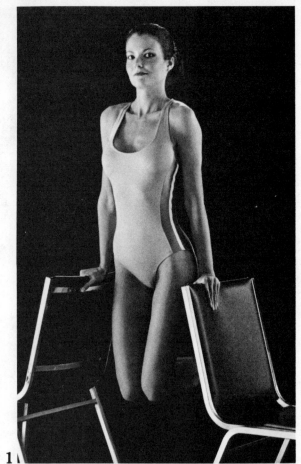

1

2

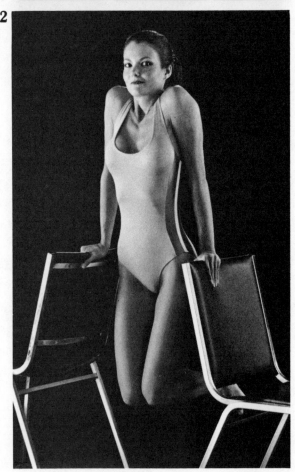

EXERCISE:
SPOON SWING

RATING: B
EQUIPMENT:
ONE TABLESPOON

Starting Position: While seated, lean face-down and insert the handle of an ordinary tablespoon between the lips. Insert the handle into the mouth just far enough to permit the lips to grasp it. Do not allow the spoon to touch the teeth.

Movement: Try to swing the spoon back and forth with the squeezing action of the lips. Repeat for one minute.

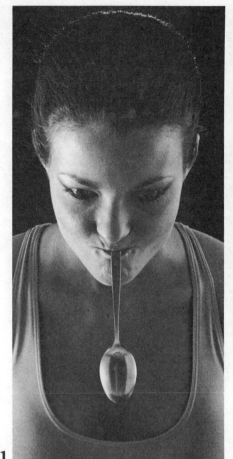

1

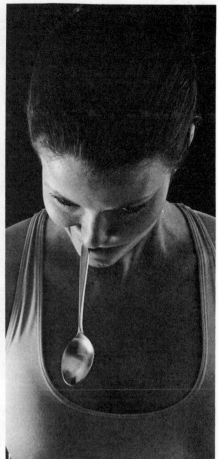

2

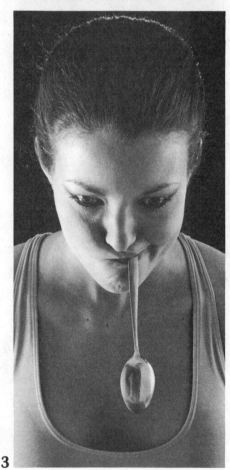

3

BODY SHAPING: FACE AND NECK

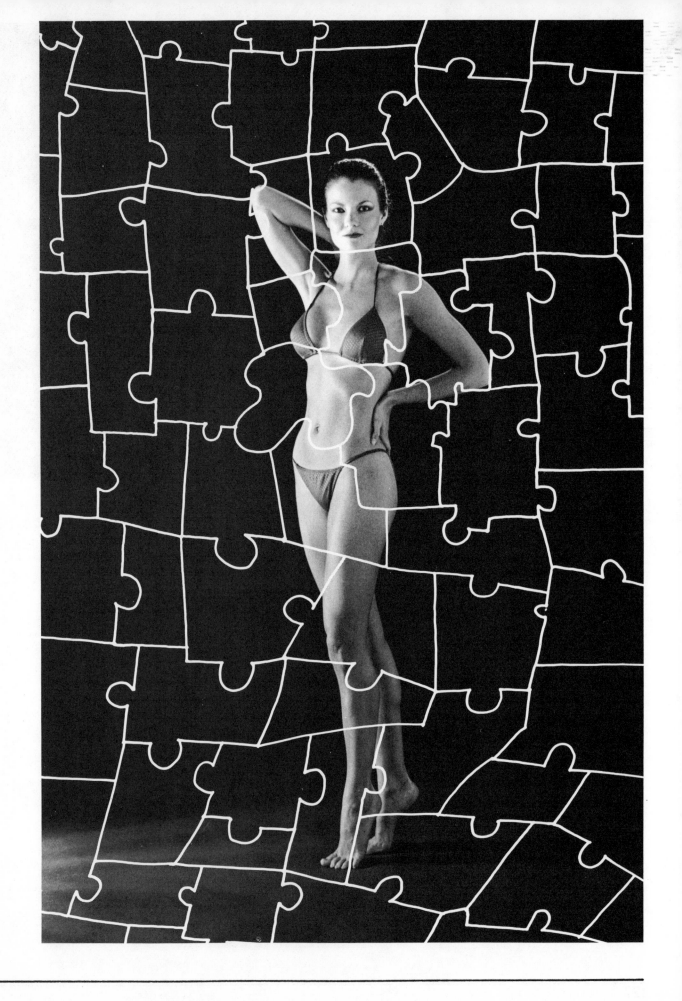

CHAPTER 12
ORGANIZ-ING A BODY-SHAPING PROGRAM

The body will tolerate only a limited amount of disproportionate training. Women who want to strengthen and shape their thighs will accomplish this more efficiently by training all the major parts of the body, not just the thighs. With this concept in mind, it is important to review the fundamental rules of body shaping.

Rules for Body Shaping

1. Perform one set of 4-6 exercises for the lower body and 6-8 exercises for the upper body. Do no more than 12 exercises in any workout.
2. Select a resistance on each exercise that allows the performance of between 8-12 repetitions.
3. Continue each exercise until no additional repetitions are possible. When 12 or more repetitions are performed, increase the resistance by approximately 5 percent at the next workout.
4. Work the largest muscles first and move quickly from one exercise to the next. This procedure develops heart-lung endurance.
5. Concentrate on flexibility by slowly stretching during the first three repetitions of each exercise.
6. Accentuate the lowering portion of each repetition.
7. Move slower, never faster, if in doubt about the

speed of movement.
8. Do everything possible to isolate and work each large muscle group to exhaustion.
9. Attempt constantly to increase the number of repetitions or the amount of weight, or both. But do not sacrifice form in an attempt to produce results.
10. Train no more than three times a week.
11. Keep accurate records -- date, resistance, repetitions, and overall training time -- of each workout.
12. Vary the workouts often.

BODY-SHAPING PROGRAMS

Application of the body-shaping rules to the Master Listing of Exercises makes it possible to organize numerous effective programs. The following programs have been used successfully by women of all ages.

CHOOSING A PROGRAM

There are 17 programs grouped into five categories: basic, change-of-pace, barbell, freehand, and negative.

The basic programs are designed to lay a

foundation of strength for all muscle groups.

Change-of-pace programs add variety to the routine of repeated exercises.

Barbell programs are usually more advanced than the basic or change-of-pace routines.

Freehand programs are specifically intended for those away from home. These exercises can be done in a motel room, on the beach, outside camping, or anywhere.

Negative programs accentuate the lowering phases of certain exercises. They offer the most intense mode of training.

Most beginners should initiate their exercises by a careful examination of Basic Programs 1, 2, and 3. These programs are specifically planned to furnish a primary level strength for all the major muscles within six weeks.

Basic Program 1 should be performed three times a week for the first two weeks. Basic Program 2 should be performed for the second two weeks, and Basic Program 3, for the third two weeks.

After the first six weeks the woman can progress to the other five basic programs. For the next six weeks, programs can be alternated according to choice. Regardless of her selection, the woman should keep accurate records of the exercises, sequence, weight, and repetitions as suggested by the charts in this chapter.

Beginning with the third six weeks, the woman should perform one negative program per week, usually on Friday or Saturday. The other two workouts should usually come from the basic group. Change-of-pace, barbell, or freehand programs, however, can be substituted for any of the basic programs.

A body-shaping program can enrich any woman's life. But it must be **proper** body shaping — body shaping properly organized and properly performed.

MASTER LISTING OF EXERCISES

BODY PART	"A" Rated	"B" Rated	"C" Rated
THIGHS	Partner Leg Curl Leaning Knee Bend One-Legged Squat Negative-Emphasized Squat with Partner Hip Adduction with Partner Chair Step-up with Plastic Bottle	Straddle Lift with Barbell Stiff-Legged Deadlift Lunge with Plastic Bottles Chair Step-up Wall Leg Press Squat Wide Squat Lunge Bent-Over One-Legged Squat Inner Thigh Squeeze Outer Thigh Squeeze	Double Leg Raise to Side Side Leg Circle Standing Thigh Raise Standing Side Leg Raise Lying Side Leg Raise Shoulder Stand Leg Scissor

MASTER LISTING OF EXERCISES

BODY PART	"A" Rated	"B" Rated	"C" Rated
CALVES	One-Legged Calf Raise with Plastic Bottle One-Legged Calf Raise Partner Foot Flexion	Calf Raise Outside Ankle Strengthening Against a Door Inside Ankle Strengthening Against a Door Seated Calf Raise Toe Curl Bent-Over Calf Raise	Toe Spread Ankle Circle
FACE AND NECK	Point the Face Nose Raise Lower Lid Close Forehead Slide Jaw Pull Web Neck Front Neck Flexion Against Hand Resistance Rear Neck Extension Against Hand Resistance Side Neck Flexion Against Hand Resistance Shoulder Shrug with Plastic Bottles	Spoon Swing Neck Rotation Against Hand Resistance Torso Shrug	
HIPS AND BUTTOCKS	Squat with Plastic Bottles One-Legged Squat Negative-Emphasized Squat with Partner Barbell Squat Chair Step-up with Plastic Bottle Hip Adduction with Partner Hip Abduction with Partner	Squat Wide Squat Wall Leg Press Lunge with Plastic Bottles Chair Step-up Reverse Leg Raise Bent-Kneed Situp with Partner Hip Extension	Standing Thigh Raise Static Chair Squeeze Static Chair Spread

BODY SHAPING: ORGANIZING A BODY-SHAPING PROGRAM

MASTER LISTING OF EXERCISES

BODY PART	"A" Rated	"B" Rated	"C" Rated
BACK	Chinup Stiff-Legged Dead Lift Bent-Armed Pullover with Plastic Bottles Straight-Armed Pullover with Cans Shoulder Shrug with Plastic Bottles	Lying Chinup Bent-Over Row with Plastic Bottles Bent-Over Row with Cans Back Hyperextension with Partner Back Hyperextension and Reverse Leg Raise Bent-Over Lateral Raise with Cans Lateral Raise with Cans	Reverse Leg Raise Back Hyperextension Bent-Over Shrug with Plastic Bottles
BUST	Standing Chair Dip Negative Chair Dip Bench Press with Barbell Bent-Armed Pullover with Barbell Bent-Armed Lateral Raise with Dumbbells Pushup Between Chairs Bent-Armed Pullover with Plastic Bottles Bench Press with Plastic Bottles	Pushup Straight-Armed Pullover with Cans Dynamic Chest Contraction Pushup on Chair Upright Row with Plastic Bottles Front Raise with Cans	Pushup on Knees Wall Press Front Raise with Plastic Bottles
WAIST	Trunk Curl Negative Trunk Curl Reverse Trunk Curl Side Bend with Plastic Bottle	V-up Side Trunk Curl Twisting Trunk Curl Twisting Reverse Trunk Curl Side Bend with Towel Side Bend	Leg Raise in Chair Chair Twist Leg Crossover Trunk Roll
UPPER ARMS	Triceps Extension with One Can Triceps Extension_ with Cans Biceps Curl with Cans Seated One-Armed Curl with Can Chinup Negative Chinup Standing Chair Dip	Overhead Press with Cans Reverse Curl with Cans Triceps Extension with Towel Lying Chinup Partner-Assisted Triceps Extension Chair-Seat Dip	Wrist Curl with Plastic Bottle Reverse Wrist Curl with Plastic Bottle Finger Curl with Plastic Bottle Newspaper Wadding

Basic Workout 1

1. Squat with Plastic Bottles p. 36
2. Partner Leg Curl p. 48
3. Wall Leg Press p. 52
4. One-Legged Calf Raise with Plastic Bottle p. 64
5. Partner Foot Flexion p. 65
6. Chinup p. 72
7. Negative Chair Dip p. 83
8. Biceps Curl with Cans p. 95
9. Triceps Extension with One Can p. 94
10. Trunk Curl p. 106
11a. Front Neck Flexion Against Hand Resistance p. 121
11b. Rear Neck Extension Against Hand Resistance p. 123
11c. Side Neck Flexion Against Hand Resistance p. 123
12. All Facial Exercises p. 119 - 122

1st two wks.

Basic Workout 2

1. One-Legged Squat p. 36
2. Hip Adduction with Partner p. 50
3. Hip Abduction with Partner p. 51
4. Partner Leg Curl p. 48
5. Leaning Knee Bend p. 48
6. One-Legged Calf Raise with Plastic Bottle p. 64
7. Stiff-Legged Deadlift p. 73
8. Pushup Between Chairs p. 65
9. Seated One-Armed Curl p. 95
10. Triceps Extension with Cans p. 94
11. Negative Trunk Curl p. 107
12. Side Bend with Plastic Bottle p. 108

2nd two weeks

BODY SHAPING: ORGANIZING A BODY-SHAPING PROGRAM

Basic Workout 3

1. Reverse Leg Raise p.42
2. Chair Step-up with Plastic Bottle p.38
3. Bent-Kneed Situp with Partner p.43
4. One-Legged Calf Raise with Plastic Bottle p.64
5. Partner Foot Flexion p.65
6. Outside Ankle Strengthening Against a Door p.66
7. Inside Ankle Strengthening Against a Door p.67 (3RD TWO WKS.)
8. Shoulder Shrug p.74
9. Bench Press with Plastic Bottles p.86
10. Chinup p.96
11. Standing Chair Dip p.97

12a. Neck Rotation Against Hand Resistance p.125
12b. Torso Shrug p.126

Basic Workout 4

1. Lunge with Plastic Bottles
2. Static Chair Squeeze
3. Static Chair Spread
4. Shoulder Stand Leg Scissor
5. Bent-Over One-Legged Squat
6. Bent-Over Calf Raise
7. Bent-Over Row with Cans
8. Bent-Armed Pullover with Plastic Bottles
9. Pushup on Knees
10. Reverse Curl with Cans
11. Partner-Assisted Triceps Extension
12. Shoulder Shrug with Plastic Bottles

Basic Workout 5

1. Chair Step-up
2. Partner Leg Curl
3. One-Legged Squat
4. Side Leg Circle
5. One-Legged Calf Raise with Plastic Bottle
6. Ankle Circle
7. Straight-Armed Pullover with Cans
8. Pushup on Chair
9. Front Raise with Cans
10a. Finger Curl with Plastic Bottle
10b. Wrist Curl with Plastic Bottle
10c. Reverse Wrist Curl with Plastic Bottle
10d. Newspaper Wadding
11. Twisting Reverse Trunk Curl
12. Torso Shrug

Basic Workout 6

1. Squat with Plastic Bottles
2. Double Leg Raise to the Side
3. Wall Leg Press
4. Seated Calf Raise
5. Bent-Over Lateral Raise with Cans
6. Bent-Over Shrug
7. Standing Chair Dip
8. Wall Press
9. Biceps Curl with Cans
10. Overhead Press with Cans
11. Side Bend
12. Chair Twist

Basic Workout 7

1. Negative-Emphasized Squat with Partner
2. Standing Side Leg Raise
3. Lying Side Leg Raise
4. Partner Leg Curl
5. Straddle Lift with Barbell
6. Toe Spread
7. Partner Foot Flexion
8. Lateral Raise with Cans
9. Overhead Press with Cans
10. Front Raise with Plastic Bottles
11. Upright Row with Plastic Bottles
12. Leg Raise in Chair

Basic Workout 8

1. Hip Adduction with Partner
2. Hip Adduction with Partner
3. One-Legged Calf Raise with Plastic Bottle
4. Barbell Squat
5. Back Hyperextension with Partner
6. Bent-Armed Lateral Raise with Dumbbells
7. Negative Chair Dip
8. Seated One-Armed Curl with Can
9. Chair-Seat Dip
10. Trunk Curl
11. Leg Crossover Trunk Roll
12a. Spoon Swing
12b. Jaw Pull
12c. Point the Face

Change-of-Pace Workout 1

1. Trunk Curl
2. Lying Chinup
3. Triceps Extension with One Can
4. Wall Press
5. Wrist Curl with Plastic Bottle
6. Chinup
7. Back Hyperextension
8. Double Leg Raise to the Side
9. Calf Raise
10. Partner Leg Curl
11. Chair Step-up with Plastic Bottle
12. Shoulder Shrug with Plastic Bottles

Change-of-Pace Workout 2

1. Trunk Curl
2. Chinup
3. One-Legged Calf Raise with Dumbbell
4. Partner Foot Flexion
5. Inside Ankle Strengthening Against a Door
6. Outside Ankle Strengthening Against a Door
7. Torso Shrug
8. Negative Chair Dip
9. Biceps Curl with Barbell
10. Negative Chinup
11. Bent-Armed Pullover with Barbell
12. Straddle Lift with Barbell

Barbell Workout 1

1. Barbell Squat
2. Partner Leg Curl
3. Stiff-Legged Deadlift
4. One-Legged Calf Raise
5. Bent-Armed Lateral Raise with Dumbbells
6. Bench Press with Barbell
7. Chinup
8. Standing Chair Dip
9. Trunk Curl
10. Reverse Trunk Curl
11a. Front Neck Flexion Against Hand Resistance
11b. Rear Neck Extension Against Hand Resistance

Barbell Workout 2

1. Hip Adduction with Partner
2. Hip Adduction with Partner
3. Leaning Knee Bend
4. Barbell Squat
5. One-Legged Calf Raise with Dumbbell
6. Bent-Over Row with Barbell
7. Chinup
8. Triceps Extension with One Dumbbell
9. Negative Chair Dip
10. Seated One Arm Curl
11. Negative Chinup
12. Side Bend with Dumbbell

Freehand Workout 1

1. Hip Extension
2. Squat
3. Outer Thigh Squeeze
4. Inner Thigh Squeeze
5. Calf Raise
6. Toe Curl
7. Reverse Leg Raise
8. Back Hyperextension
9. Pushup
10. Lying Chinup
11. V-up
12. Neck Rotation Against Hand Resistance

Freehand Workout 2

1. Wide Squat
2. Lunge
3. Standing Thigh Raise
4. Calf Raise
5. Back Hyperextension and Reverse Leg Raise
6. Dynamic Chest Contraction
7. Lying Chinup
8. Triceps Extension with Towel
9. Twisting Trunk Curl
10. Side Trunk Curl
11. Side Neck Flexion Against Hand Resistance
12a. Jaw Pull
12b. Web Neck
12c. Lower Lid Close

Freehand Workout 3

1. Hip Adduction with Partner
2. Hip Abduction with Partner
3. Negative-Emphasized Squat with Partner
4. Partner Leg Curl
5. Wall Leg Press
6. Partner Foot Flexion
7. One-Legged Calf Raise
8. Lying Chinup
9. Trunk Curl
10. Side Bend with Towel
11a. Front Neck Flexion Against Resistance
11b. Rear Neck Extension Against Resistance
12a. Nose Raise
12b. Point the Face
12c. Forehead Slide

Negative Workout 1

1. Negative-Emphasized Squat with Partner
2. Partner Leg Curl
3. One-Legged Calf Raise with Plastic Bottle
4. Back Hyperextension with Partner
5. Bent-Armed Pullover with Plastic Bottles
6. Negative Chinup
7. Bent-Armed Lateral Raise with Dumbbells
8. Negative Chair Dip
9. Negative Trunk Curl
10a. Neck Rotation Against Hand Resistance
10b. Front Neck Flexion Against Hand Resistance
10c. Rear Neck Extension Against Hand Resistance
11. Shoulder Shrug with Plastic Bottles

Negative Workout 2

1. Stiff-Legged Deadlift
2. Negative Trunk Curl
3. Pushup
4. Negative Chinup
5. Negative Chair Dip
6. One-Legged Calf Raise
7. Leaning Knee Bend
8. Negative-Emphasized Squat with Partner
9. Torso Shrug
10a. Front Neck Flexion Against Hand Resistance Performed in a Negative Fashion
10b. Rear Neck Extension Against Hand Resistance Performed in a Negative Fashion

BODY SHAPING: ORGANIZING A BODY-SHAPING PROGRAM

BODY-SHAPING PROGRESS CHART

BASIC WORKOUT I —

NAME

DATE

BODYWEIGHT

	EXERCISE								
S **E** **Q** **U** **E** **N** **C** **E**	1	Squat with Plastic Bottles							
	2	Partner Leg Curl							
	3	Wall Leg Press							
	4	One-Legged Calf Raise with Plastic Bottle							
	5	Partner Foot Flexion							
	6	Chinup							
	7	Negative Chair Dip							
	8	Biceps Curl with Cans							
	9	Triceps Extension with One Can							
	10	Trunk Curl							
	11a 11b 11c	Front Neck Flexion Against Hand Resistance Rear Neck Extension Against Hand Resistance Side Neck Flexion Against Hand Resistance							
	12	All Facial Exercises							

BODY-SHAPING PROGRESS CHART
BASIC WORKOUT 2

NAME _____

DATE _____

BODYWEIGHT

EXERCISE							
S 1	One-Legged Squat						
E 2	Hip Adduction with Partner						
Q 3	Hip Abduction with Partner						
U 4	Partner Leg Curl						
E 5	Leaning Knee Bend						
N 6	One-Legged Calf Raise with Plastic Bottle						
C 7	Stiff-Legged Deadlift						
E 8	Pushup Between Chairs						
9	Seated One-Armed Curl						
10	Triceps Extension with Cans						
11	Negative Trunk Curl						
12	Side Bend with Plastic Bottle						

BODY-SHAPING PROGRESS CHART
BASIC WORKOUT 3

NAME _____

DATE _____

BODYWEIGHT _____

	EXERCISE									
S	1	Reverse Leg Raise								
E	2	Chair Step-up with Plastic Bottle								
Q	3	Bent-Kneed Situp with Partner								
U	4	One-Legged Calf Raise with Bottle								
E	5	Partner Foot Flexion								
N	6	Outside Ankle Strengthening Against a Door								
C	7	Inside Ankle Strengthening Against a Door								
E	8	Shoulder Shrug								
	9	Bench Press with Plastic Bottles								
	10	Chinup								
	11	Standing Chair Dip								
	12a	Neck Rotation Against Hand Resistance								
	12b	Torso Shrug								

BODY-SHAPING PROGRESS CHART   NAME

DATE

BODYWEIGHT

EXERCISE

S E Q U E N C E

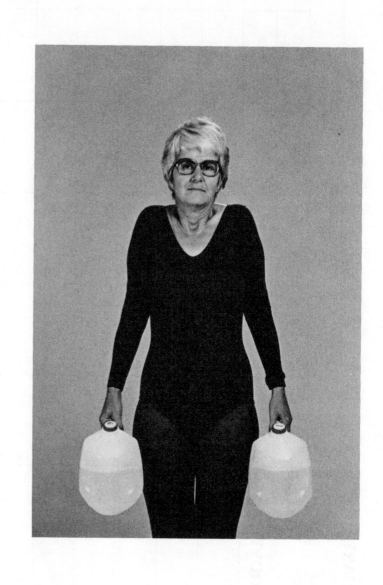

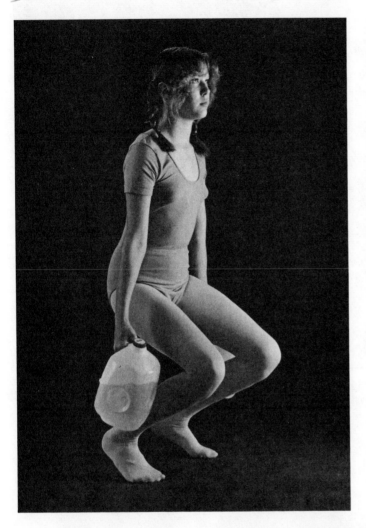

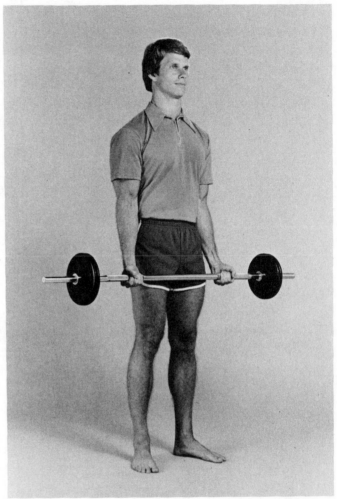

III. SPECIAL CONSIDER- ATIONS

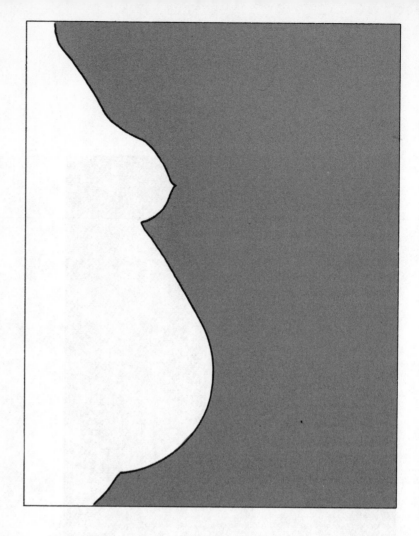

CHAPTER 13
PREGNANT WOMEN

A pregnant woman's life need not be a period of passive waiting. The opposite should be true.

The mother-to-be, whether it is for the first or the fifth time, should be in the best of health in order to enjoy her normal recreational endeavors and continue her daily activities. This is the time when a woman should pay the most attention to exercise.

There are many good reasons why exercise is important during pregnancy. All of them center on the basic relationship between exercise and muscle. Exercise, properly performed, increases strength and endurance of the muscles. It improves the tone and flexibility of the muscles, and promotes heart-lung efficiency.

Birth involves the relaxation and contraction of many major muscle groups, the uterus, abdominal, buttock, and thigh. With these muscles in good condition, the woman will have an easier time at birth. Also, she will feel and look better before and after the baby is born.

Prior to birth, especially during the last trimester, there is extra stress and strain on certain muscles. Toward the end of pregnancy, many women tilt their pelvic area forward and bend the upper part of their bodies backward to compensate for the weight of the heavy uterus. As a result, backache frequently develops. As the breasts become larger, additional stress is placed on the underlying support muscles — the pectoralis majors, the deltoids, and the trapezius.

The increasing needs of the growing fetus put an added burden on the mother's heart. Proper exercise can significantly increase the heart's efficiency.

There is slowing of blood flow in the lower extremities during pregnancy. Many times this can cause stagnation of the blood in the legs, which leads to varicose veins. Exercise will improve circulation.

Pregnancy often disturbs the gastrointestinal tract. This can result in constipation and hemorrhoids. Proper exercise can assist by providing tone and massage to the intestinal tract.

Exercise causes the body to burn calories at a higher than normal rate. A pregnant woman can consume more nutritious food and still not add excess body fat.

If a women establishes sensible exercise habits during pregnancy, they will carry over into her everyday life style. These habits should provide positive examples for her children to follow.

Both the mother and the children should know the importance of muscles and how they work.

The body contains three types of muscles: the voluntary or skeletal muscles, the involuntary muscles such as those of the digestive tract, and the heart muscle.

The skeletal muscles are composed of 250 million small fibers, and they make up 32 percent of the bodyweight of the typical American female.

Muscles are arranged in pairs. One set of muscles is on one side for the purpose of bending at the

SPECIAL CONSIDERATIONS

joint. Another set of muscles is on the opposite side of the same joint to straighten it. A simple example of this paired action is the muscles of the upper arm which serve the purpose of bending and straightening the arm at the joint of the elbow. The muscles in the front of the elbow joint, primarily the biceps, bend the arm. The muscles in the rear of the elbow, the triceps, straighten it.

Similar situations exist on both sides of all human joints, although many are more complex than the muscles involved in movement around the elbow joint.

Depending on the desired direction of movement at the moment, these opposite-working sets of muscles are called either agonist or antagonist muscles. An agonist muscle produces movement by contraction. An antagonist muscle limits or stops movement by refusing to permit itself to be stretched.

In order for movement to occur, an agonist muscle must reduce its length with a pulling force that produces movement. But simultaneously, the antagonist muscle must permit movement, by allowing its length to be increased. During all movements, while one set of muscles is getting shorter, another set of muscles must be getting longer.

Muscles produce movement by synchronized contraction and relaxation.

In much the same way, the birth process, although partially controlled by hormones and involuntary muscles, is still greatly assisted by the strength and flexibility of the skeletal muscles. During labor and delivery, most muscles of the woman's body work to capacity.

Proper exercise helps a pregnant woman to improve her ability to contract and relax her muscles.

Exercise: What Kind? How Much?

While pregnancy and birth involve most muscle groups to some degree, the primary muscles affected are the midsection, hip, lower back, and chest. Special attention should be given these areas. But at the same time, other groups of muscles such as the thighs, calves, shoulders, upper back, and arms should not be neglected.

One recommended group of body-shaping and strengthening exercises is as follows:
1. Wide squat
2. Hip extension
3. Bent-kneed situp with partner
4. Static chair squeeze
5. Static chair spread
6. Calf raise
7. Straight-armed pullover with cans
8. Bench press with cans
9. Biceps curl with cans
10. Shoulder shrug with plastic bottles
11. Trunk curl
12. Side bend with plastic bottle

A pregnant woman should begin by performing one set of 8 repetitions of each of the 12 movements. She should exercise every other day, or three times a week, and add a repetition each day until 12 are reached. When 12 repetitions can be performed in correct style, she should add several pounds of resistance and reduce the repetitions to 8.

Questions and Answers
About Pregnancy and Exercise

Q. Will a regular exercise program make child birth easier?
A. To answer this question with a **yes** requires nothing more than common sense, according to Dr. Clayton Thomas. "If you could separate all the people on earth into those who exercise and those who do not, who do you think would be the healthiest and have the easiest time having babies? It would be a paradox if the sedentary person had fewer problems. I know of no evidence that exercise is harmful in pregnancy."

Q. Should a woman athlete discontinue competition during pregnancy?
A. Noticeable changes in athletic performances first show up at the end of the third month. Most mothers gain only about three pounds in the first trimester, but in the second trimester, the uterus

expands 20 times, and a woman will gain about 10 pounds. This extra weight, a protruding abdomen, a loss of balance, and the effects of water retention and anemia, may simply make sports competition too complicated. Even the well-trained athlete will find it difficult to do her best at this point.

Because of the deterioration in performance most athletes give up competition but not exercise by the third month. A woman who is used to competition and heavy training could safely compete beyond this time. Physicians get a bit alarmed when they hear of these efforts and recommend that athletes stop competition by the sixth month of pregnancy. But there is no concrete evidence that competition during pregnancy is harmful, and a woman should judge when it is time to quit by the way she feels.

Q. Will having a baby ruin athletic ability?
A. Considering the number of mothers who have broken world records and won prizes in major competitions, it is difficult to imagine how many people still believe the myth that having a baby will ruin an athlete. Madeline Manning won a gold medal in the 800 meters in the 1968 Olympics, got married and had a baby, then broke her record in the 1972 games. In 1971, the professional tennis star Margaret Court announced she was leaving the tennis circuit until after the birth of her first child. Most followers thought she was finished as a tennis star. The next year, following the birth of her baby, she won 23 out of 26 tournaments and over $200,000 to become one of the highest female money winners of all time.

Q. Exactly what is a miscarriage? Is there danger of miscarriage if a woman competes in vigorous sports?
A. A miscarriage means that the fetus is born before it is capable of surviving outside the mother's body. The majority of miscarriages occur during the second or third month of pregnancy while a small number carry through to the seventh month. In microscopic examinations of miscarried embryos and fetuses, more than 80 percent reveal a deformity or biological malfunction that would make them unable to survive and live a normal life. A miscarriage, in

most instances, should be considered one of nature's own built-in controls. Any unusual bleeding from the vagina, however, should be reported to a physician.

There is very little danger of miscarriage from vigorous sport participation, especially if the woman is accustomed to the activity. The fetus is well-cushioned. It floats in a sack of fluid that works like a shock absorber. A pregnant woman cannot jiggle a baby loose by running, jumping, or horseback riding. Nor can she harm it by swimming. Very strong stomach blows or falls in the eighth or ninth month might start labor contractions prematurely. Physicians, therefore, advise against vigorous or contact sports toward the end of pregnancy.

Q. What type of exercise program should a woman follow after her baby is born?
A. Unless a physician advises the mother otherwise, or barring unusual complications, she may begin a simple exercise while she is in the hospital. Light movements should be performed daily, once or twice at first, with gradual increases in repetitions. A description of her first week of exercise might be as follows:
Leg raise and tuck. Lie flat on the back. Keeping the left leg straight, raise the right foot off the bed about 6 inches. Smoothly bend the right knee, then straighten, and lower. Do the same with the left leg.

After the first week of performing this simple exercise, she can begin some of the freehand movements that she became accustomed to during pregnancy.

Suggested exercises would be the squat, pullover, calf raise, and negative-accentuated trunk curl.

She should do them daily, with gradual increases in repetitions, for the next two weeks.

By the end of the third week, she may begin some lighting walking and add harder exercises to her routine.

Approximately four weeks after the baby is born,

SPECIAL CONSIDERATIONS: PREGNANT WOMEN

the woman should be ready to return to her previous routine, resistance exercises every other day, with brisk walking in between.

After a baby is born, the average woman spends at least six weeks resting before getting back into her routine. Most well-conditioned women are able to start training in four weeks.

Q. Does every pregnant woman get stretch marks? How can they be prevented?
A. Stretch marks are caused by the tearing of the elastic tissues in the skin that accompanies enlargement of breasts, distention of the abdomen, and the deposition of subcutaneous fat. They are pink or purplish-red lines during pregnancy. The lines become permanent grayish-white scarlike marks after delivery. Some women never develop stretch marks despite bearing several children. Others lose most of the tone in their skin after one pregnancy. Evidently there is an inherited factor involved in stretch marks.

Stretch marks cannot be considered evidence that a woman has borne a child, however, because they sometimes are seen in women who have never been pregnant.

Once a woman gets stretch marks, there is nothing she can do about them. She might help to prevent them by making sure she does not gain excessive amounts of body fat and that she adheres to a well-balanced diet.

Q. How are varicose veins related to pregnancy?
A. Varicose veins are bulging, twisted, and knotted veins that are usually located right under the skin. While they frequently occur in pregnant women, they also appear in other women and men as well. Most often they develop in the legs, although they can pop out in other places. When they appear in the anal area, they are called hemorrhoids. Their presence is due to two factors: One, many pregnancies contribute to a generally weakened condition of the veins in the legs if the pressure created by the baby cuts off some circulation. Two, varicose veins can be inherited. In such a case, the individual probably inherited a tendency to inelasticity in the walls of the veins.

In both instances, however, the results are the same: there is a weakness or malfunction within the flaplike valves of the vein. As the weight of the blood on the vein wall increases, the vein bulges. After continuous stretching it loses its elasticity.

Q. Will exercise help varicose veins?
A. Yes. Any type of contracting or pumping of the leg muscles helps to milk the blood out of the calves and thighs and propel it upward toward the heart. Brisk walking is good exercise. Calf raises and squats are even better. All women can benefit by maintaining muscle tone in the thigh and calf muscles. The strong, firm muscles around the deep veins help provide external support and help protect them from overstretching and damage.

Q. Can varicose veins be prevented?
A. If a woman has inherited a tendency toward varicose veins, she probably will not be able to prevent them. The following precautionary measures, however, may help prevent or minimize them:
• Do not stand for long periods of time. If this cannot be avoided, wear lightweight support stockings. When standing on a bus, at a job, or at a kitchen sink, flex the toes every few minutes and then rise slowly on the tiptoes.
• Do not sit for long periods, especially with the legs crossed. When sitting, elevate the legs or change their position. On long train, plane, or bus rides, walk about every half hour or so. On long car trips, switch drivers frequently or stop to do some light exercise every hour if possible.
• Avoid tight garments that constrict the legs: girdles, garters, and knee-high stockings. High boots with tight elastic around the top are especially damaging.
• Keep body weight within the normal range.

Q. Are there ways to keep varicose veins from getting worse?
A. Use the precautionary measures listed above in addition to the following:
• Wear support stockings. They counteract the pressure of the blood against the vein walls.
• Elevate the legs at least twice daily for 30 minutes with one or two pillows under the calves so that the legs are above the level of the heart. Be sure the knees are bent.

• Be especially careful to avoid bumping, bruising, or scratching the legs. They may cause phlebitis.
• Take long walks and exercise regularly. When walking briskly, wear support stockings.

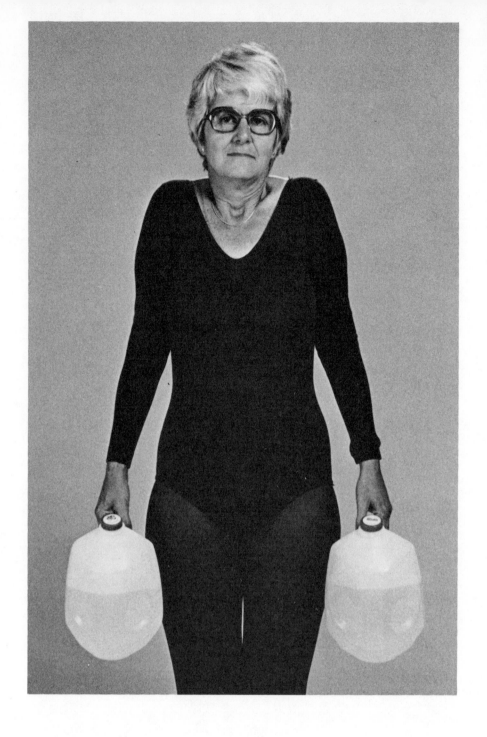

CHAPTER 14
OVER-65 AGE GROUP

The Census Bureau has estimated that there are 25 million people living in the United States over the age of 65. If present birth trends continue, an estimated 17 percent of the population will be past 65 by the year 2030. The percentage now is 10.5. By 2030, more than 50 million Americans will be 65 or older.

Physical fitness can certainly improve life for those over 65. For those with normal health there is no better exercise than proper strength training and body shaping.

There are a few people in this age group, however, who should be precluded from vigorous exercise. Exercise may aggravate the condition of those who have acute arthritis, anemia, tuberculosis, severe kidney or liver diseases, or severe heart problems. In these cases, a physician's recommendations should be rigidly adhered to.

A complete medical examination should, of course, be a prerequisite for anyone over 65 who is interested in exercise.

The following 12 exercises are an example of an effective grouping of body-shaping exercises for older women. The movements should be performed exactly as listed and described.

1. Wide squat between chairs
2. Lying leg raises
3. Ankle circle
4. Pushup on knees
5. Shoulder shrug with plastic bottles
6. Overhead press with cans
7. Biceps curl with cans
8. Trunk curl
9. Side bend with plastic bottle
10. Chair twist
11. Newspaper wadding
12. Face exercise

SPECIAL CONSIDERATIONS

EXERCISE:
JAW PULL

RATING: A
EQUIPMENT:
NONE

Starting Position: Drop the lower jaw by relaxing it. Hook three fingers behind and upon the lower teeth.

Movement: Pull the lower jaw down further. Close the jaw slowly, without clamping fingers, and then stretch against the resistance provided by the fingers and hand.
Hint: Do not stick out the neck; keep it in line with the spine. Extension of the neck prevents isolation in the exercise.

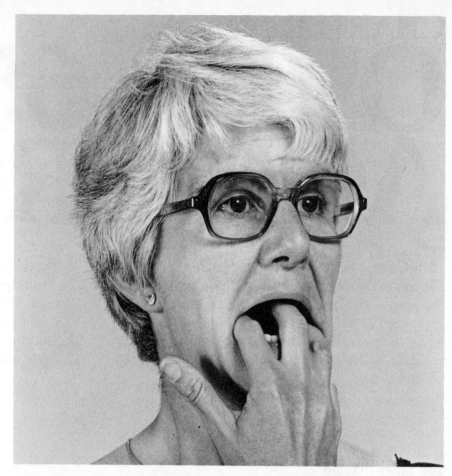

EXERCISE:
BICEPS CURL
WITH CANS

RATING: A
EQUIPMENT:
TWO CANS

Starting Position: Grasp a can in each hand with the palms up. Stand erect.

Movement: While keeping the body straight, smoothly curl the cans. Slowly lower and repeat.

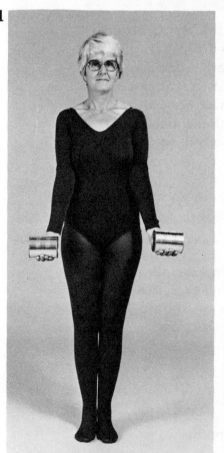

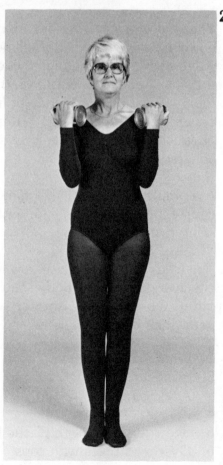

EXERCISE:
POINT THE FACE

RATING: A
EQUIPMENT:
NONE

Starting Position: Stand in front of a mirror.

Movement: Try to make the eyes, nose, chin, and cheeks squeeze to a point in the center of the face. Be sure to pucker the lips, flatten the chin, and wrinkle the bridge of the nose. Squeeze, pause, release, and repeat.

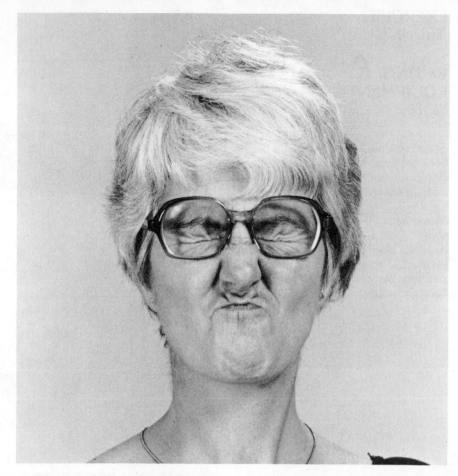

EXERCISE:
SIDE BEND WITH PLASTIC BOTTLE

RATING: A
EQUIPMENT:
WATER-FILLED PLASTIC BOTTLE

Starting Position: Grasp bottle in right hand and stand erect. Place left hand on top of head.

Movement: Bend to the right side as far as possible. Return to the vertical position and repeat. Change hands and work left side.

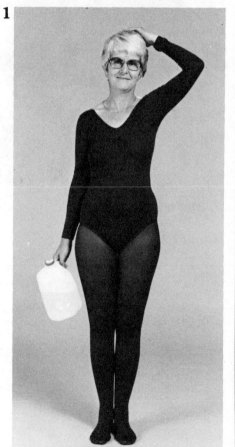
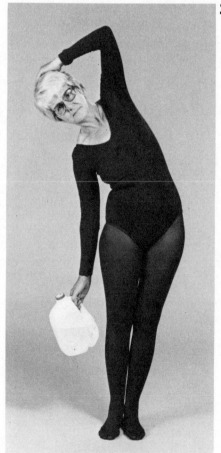

SPECIAL CONSIDERATIONS: OVER-65 AGE GROUP

EXERCISE:
TRUNK CURL

RATING: A
EQUIPMENT:
NONE

Starting Position: Lie face-up on the floor with the hands behind the head. Bring the heels close to the buttocks and spread the knees.

Movement: Try to curl the trunk to a sitting position. Only one third of a standard situp can be performed in this fashion. Pause in the contracted position. Slowly lower the trunk to the floor and repeat.

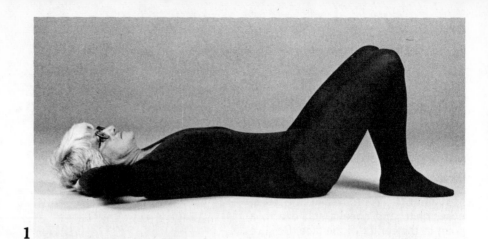

1

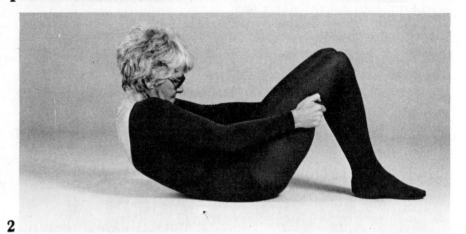

2

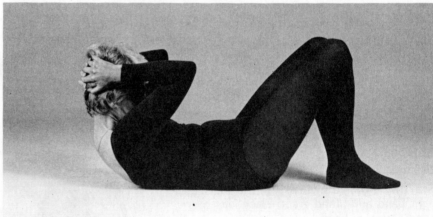

3

EXERCISE:
SHOULDER SHRUG WITH PLASTIC BOTTLES

RATING: A
EQUIPMENT:
TWO WATER-FILLED PLASTIC BOTTLES

Starting Position: Grasp the bottles and stand.

Movement: Keeping the arms straight, smoothly shrug the shoulders as high as possible. Pause in the top position. Slowly lower and repeat.

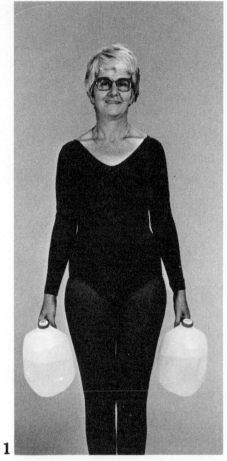

1

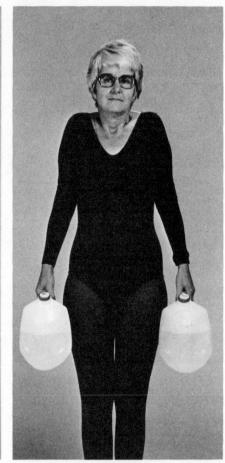

2

EXERCISE:
OVERHEAD PRESS WITH CANS

RATING: B
EQUIPMENT:
UNOPENED CANS

Starting Position: Grasp a can in each hand and bring them to the shoulders.

Movement: Press the cans overhead and lower slowly back to the shoulders. Repeat.

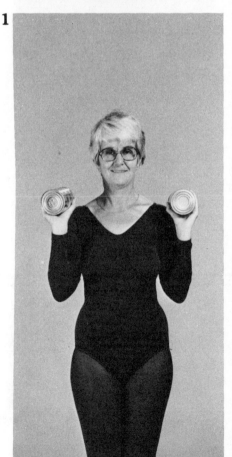

1

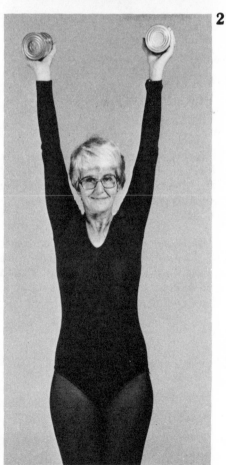

2

SPECIAL CONSIDERATIONS: OVER-65 AGE GROUP

EXERCISE:
WIDE SQUAT BETWEEN CHAIRS

RATING: B
EQUIPMENT:
TWO CHAIRS

Starting Position: Place the feet twice shoulder-width apart and turn the toes outward. Stand erect with the heels flat. Rest the hands on the chairs for balance.

Movement: Lower the body by bending the knees as far as possible. Keep the back vertical. Return to starting position and repeat. **Do not** bounce or relax at the bottom of the movement.

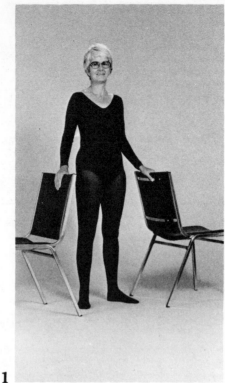

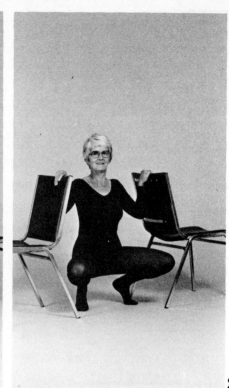

EXERCISE:
CHAIR TWIST

RATING: C
EQUIPMENT:
CHAIR

Starting Position: Sit in a chair. The left hand holds the right upper edge of the chair. The right hand holds the other edge. Both elbows should be down.

Movement: Press with the left hand, pull with the right, and gently twist the torso to the left. Hold the stretched position for about 15 seconds. Change positions to stretch the right side.

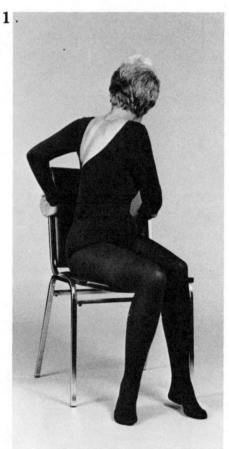

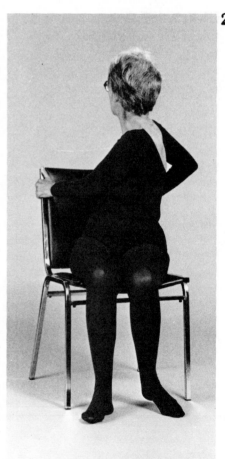

EXERCISE:
PUSHUP ON KNEES

RATING: C
EQUIPMENT:
NONE

Starting Position: Lie face-down with the palms of the hands directly under the shoulders with the arms bent.

Movement: Slowly push the body to arms' length while remaining on the knees. Lower to the floor and repeat.

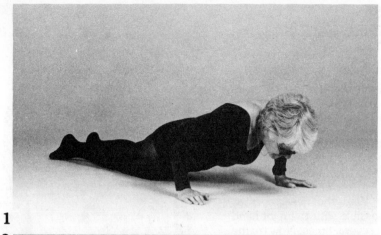

1

2

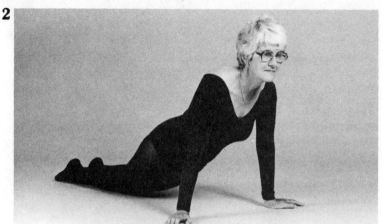

EXERCISE:
ANKLE CIRCLE

RATING: C
EQUIPMENT:
CHAIR

Starting Position: Sit in a chair and cross the left leg over the right.

Movement: Perform circular motions with the left foot. Repeat for one minute. Change feet.

1

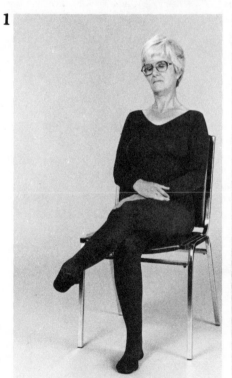

2

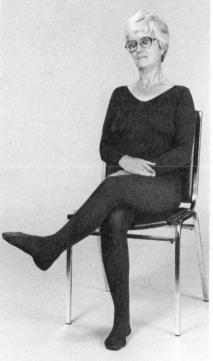

SPECIAL CONSIDERATIONS: OVER-65 AGE GROUP

EXERCISE:
NEWSPAPER WADDING

RATING: C
EQUIPMENT:
SHEETS OF NEWSPAPER

Starting Position: Stand erect. Grasp the middle of a full-size sheet of newspaper.

Movement: Wad the newspaper as quickly as possible with the right hand only. Repeat several times. Now try the left hand.

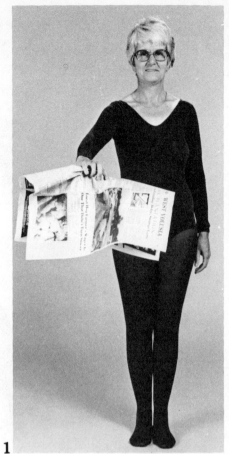

1

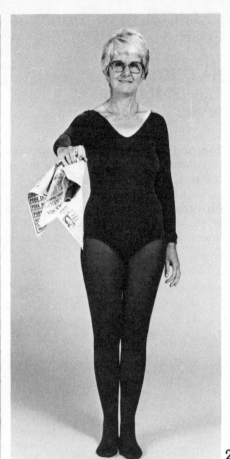

2

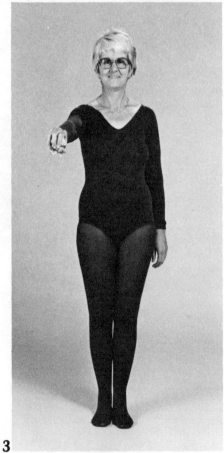

3

EXERCISE:
LYING LEG RAISE

RATING: C
EQUIPMENT:
NONE

Starting Position: Lie on the back flat on the floor.

Movement: Raise the legs to the chest with knees bent, then lower. Repeat. This movement can be performed with both legs simultaneously or one leg at a time.

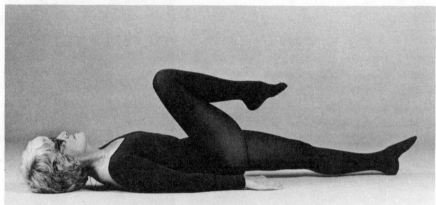

1

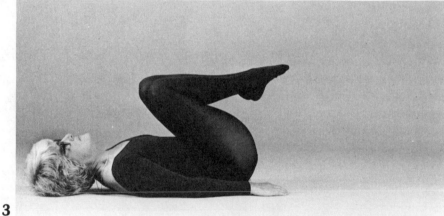

2

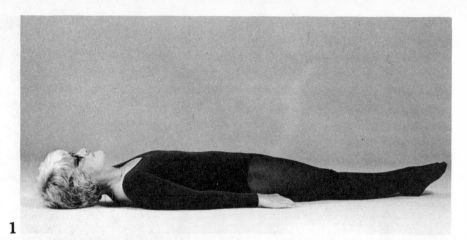

3

SPECIAL CONSIDERATIONS: OVER-65 AGE GROUP

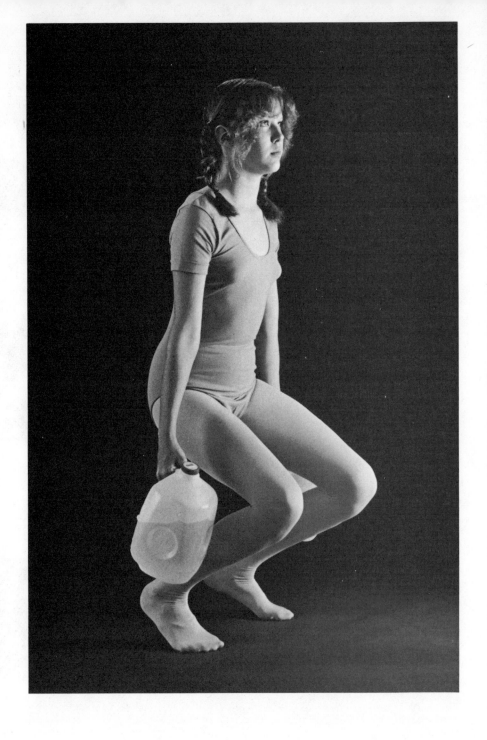

CHAPTER 15
10 TO 14 AGE GROUP

A properly conducted body-shaping and strength-training program produces the following results for the 10 to 14 age group:
1. Increased muscular strength
2. Stronger ligaments, tendons, and connective tissue
3. Improved flexibility
4. Stronger bones
5. Increased heart-lung efficiency
6. Better protection against injury
7. Improved coordination
8. Faster speed of movement

Strength training of both boys and girls before puberty, and girls after puberty, produces little muscular development. The dominant muscle-building hormone, testosterone, is not secreted in large enough amounts in girls to affect growth. Large muscular size from exercise is only possible in males after puberty.

Prior to age 10, most children will profit more by learning and practicing basic movement skills, such as throwing, kicking, tumbling, climbing, jumping, and swinging. After the age of 10, however, properly conducted body shaping will benefit all children.

Basically, the same body-shaping principles that have been used successfully with mature individuals apply to the 10 to 14 age group. It is very important that the young pay special attention to correct form in all exercises. For them supervision is very necessary.

Children under 5 feet in height and weighing less than 100 pounds should build a basic level of strength with freehand exercises before progressing to barbells. The following freehand routine is recommended as a starter program:

1. Squat with plastic bottles
2. Reverse leg raise
3. Chair step-up
4. One-legged calf raise
5. Pushup or dip between chairs
6. Shoulder shrug with plastic bottles
7. Triceps extension with cans
8. Biceps curl with cans or chinup
9. Side bend with plastic bottles
10. Trunk curl

The young should start out by performing 8 repetitions of each exercise in good form. If that seems impossible on some movements, especially the chinup, dip or even the pushup, the following variations may be made.

In the chinup, an adolescent can use her legs to help get her chin over the bar. She should place a wooden box in front of the chinning bar, step on the box, and put her chin over the bar. She should remove her feet and lower herself very slowly in 6-8 seconds then climb back and repeat. This is excellent exercise for arm and back muscles. For building shape and strength the lowering portion of the exercise is far more important than the raising part.

In pushups, the adolescent can use her knees and lower back to help straighten her arms. She should then slowly bend her arms until her chest touches the floor.

165

The squat can be done in one of two ways. The girl can bend her legs very slowly and smoothly then stand up and repeat. She can work up to 10-15 seconds lowering time on this exercise. Or, she can lower her body on one leg, stand up on two legs, and lower again on the opposite leg. Some girls may need a chair to hold to for balance. For best results from these movements, only one set of 8-12 repetitions three times a week should be done.

EXERCISE:
SQUAT WITH
PLASTIC BOTTLES

RATING: A
EQUIPMENT:
WATER-FILLED
PLASTIC BOTTLES

Starting Position: Stand erect, feet shoulder-width apart, with a bottle in each hand. The feet should be flat if working the back is desired. The heels should be elevated if working the calves is preferable.

Movement: Slowly lower the upper body by bending the knees and hips. Look straight ahead or slightly upward during the movement. Continue downward until the thighs come into contact with the backs of the calves. **Do not** relax or bounce at the bottom of the movement. Return smoothly to the starting position and repeat.

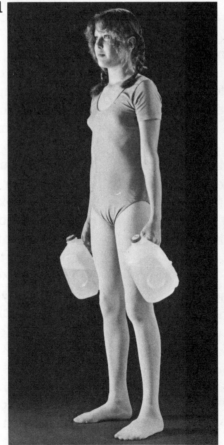

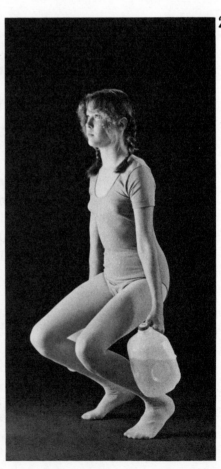

EXERCISE:
ONE-LEGGED
CALF RAISE

RATING: A
EQUIPMENT:
MINIMUM THREE-INCH
BLOCK OR STEP
AND CHAIR

Starting Position: Place the ball of the left foot on the edge of a block or stair step. Lock the knees and suspend the other foot. Balance the body by grasping a chair or stair rail.

Movement: While the knee remains locked, raise the heel as high as possible, then lower slowly to a deep stretch. Repeat until fatigued. Follow the same procedure for the right calf.

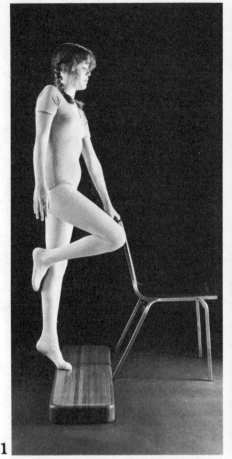

1

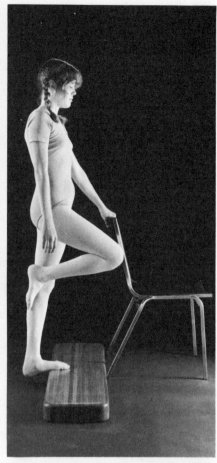

2

EXERCISE:
SHOULDER SHRUG WITH
PLASTIC BOTTLES

RATING: A
EQUIPMENT:
TWO WATER-FILLED
PLASTIC BOTTLES

Starting Position: Grasp the bottles and stand.

Movement: Keeping the arms straight, smoothly shrug the shoulders as high as possible. Pause in the top position. Slowly lower and repeat.

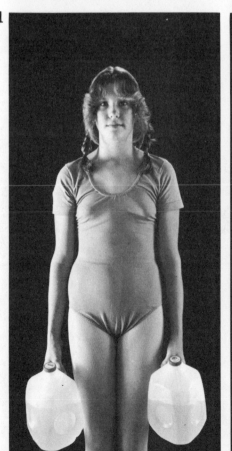

1

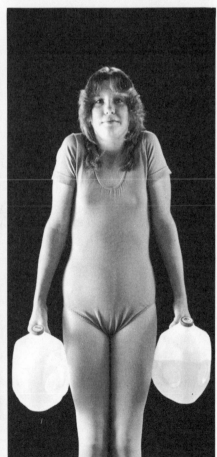

2

167

EXERCISE:
TRICEPS EXTENSION WITH CAN

RATING: A
EQUIPMENT:
ONE LARGE UNOPENED CAN

Starting Position: Hold a large can in the middle with both hands and raise it overhead. Keep the elbows by the ears.

Movement: Slowly bend and straighten the arms. Do not move the elbows. Repeat.

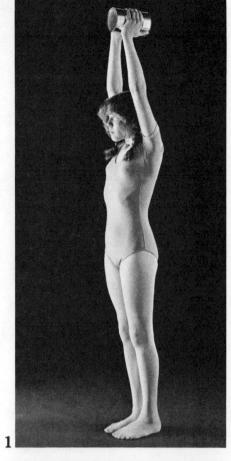

1

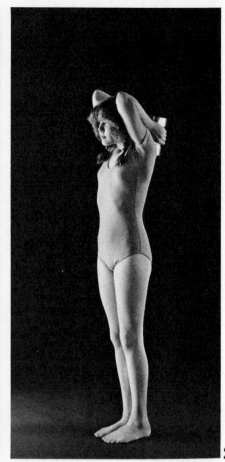

2

EXERCISE:
BICEPS CURL WITH CANS

RATING: A
EQUIPMENT:
TWO CANS

Starting Position: Grasp a can in each hand with the palms up. Stand erect.

Movement: While keeping the body straight, smoothly curl the cans. Slowly lower and repeat.

1

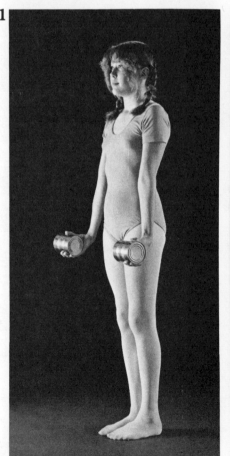

2

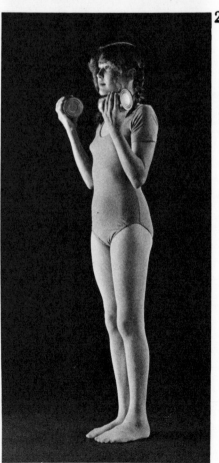

EXERCISE:
SIDE BEND WITH PLASTIC BOTTLE

RATING: A
EQUIPMENT:
WATER-FILLED PLASTIC BOTTLE

Starting Position: Grasp bottle in right hand and stand erect. Place left hand on top of head.

Movement: Bend to the right side as far as possible. Return to the vertical position and repeat. Change hands and work left side.

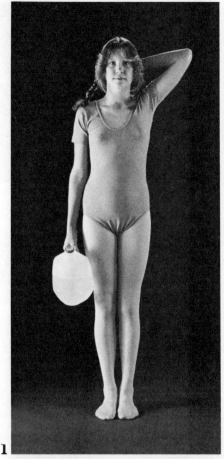 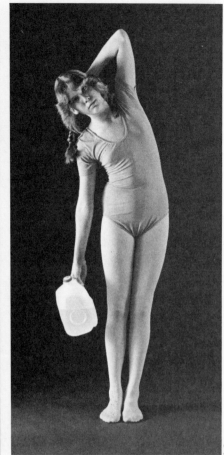

1   2

EXERCISE:
TRUNK CURL

RATING: A
EQUIPMENT:
NONE

Starting Position: Lie face-up on the floor with the hands behind the head. Bring the knees up close to the buttocks and spread the knees.

Movement: Try to curl the trunk to a sitting position. Only one-third of a standard situp can be performed in this fashion. Pause in the contracted position. Slowly lower the trunk to the floor and repeat.

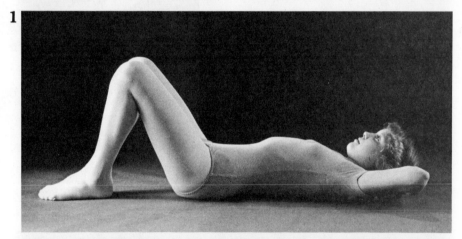

1

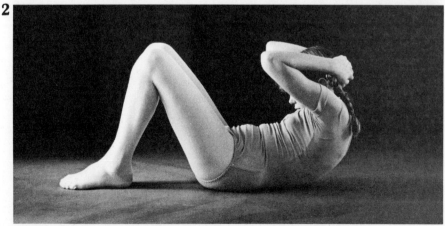

2

EXERCISE:
REVERSE LEG RAISE

RATING: B
EQUIPMENT:
NONE

Starting Position: Lie face-down on the floor. The hands should be by the hips.

Movement: Lift both legs backward as high as possible. Pause briefly at the highest position and strongly squeeze the buttocks together. Slowly return the legs to the floor and repeat.

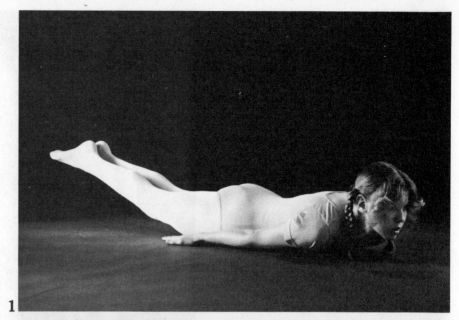

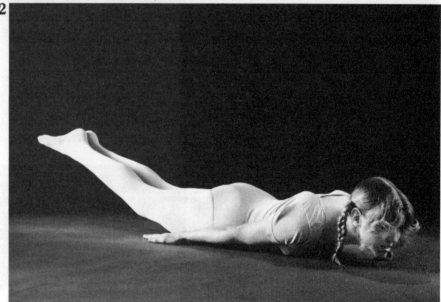

EXERCISE:
CHAIR STEP-UP

RATING: B
EQUIPMENT:
CHAIR

Starting Position: Stand erect with the left foot planted firmly in a straight-bottomed chair and the other foot on the floor.

Movement: Slowly step up on the chair, then step down with the same leg until it is completely fatigued. Switch sides and step up with the other leg.

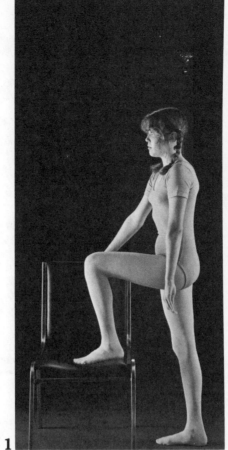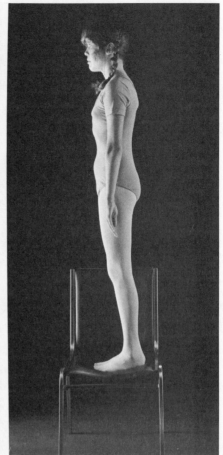

EXERCISE:
PUSHUP

RATING: B
EQUIPMENT:
NONE

Starting Position: Lie face-down on the floor with bodyweight supported on the palms of the hands and the toes. The toes should be bent and the hands should be directly under the shoulders with the arms bent.

Movement: Keeping the body straight and rigid, slowly push it to arms' length, then lower. Repeat.

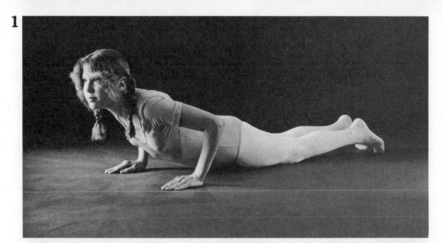

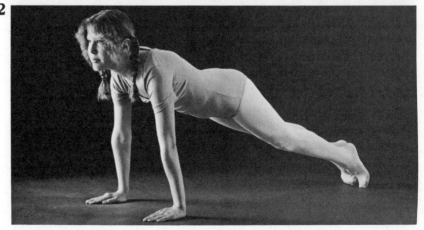

SPECIAL CONSIDERATIONS: 10 to 14 AGE GROUP

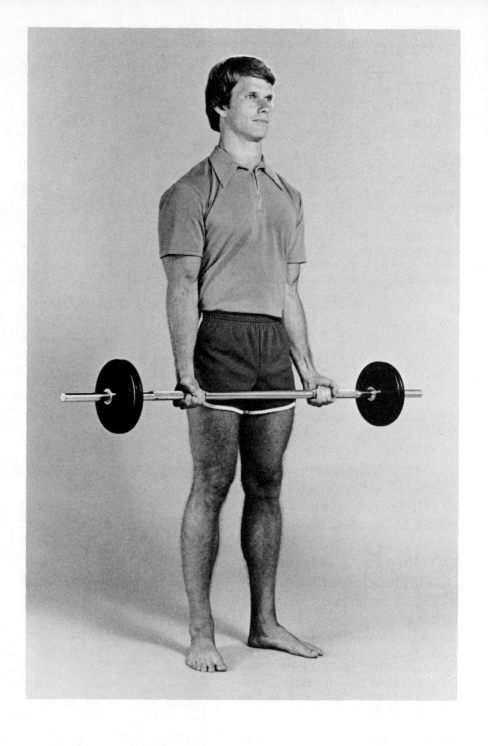

CHAPTER 16
MEN

Physical strength has been admired and envied by men since the beginning of time. Primitive tribes frequently selected the strongman as their leader. Occasionally, extraordinary muscular size and strength occurred naturally in certain men as a result of heredity or a chance mutation. But usually this size and strength was a result of intensive training. Although these men did not lift barbells, they did lift rocks, trees, and even animals.

Records of strength contests date back to ancient Greece. The most famous of all Greek athletes was probably Milo of Crotona, who lived about 540 B.C. Milo developed his strength by lifting a growing calf each day until it weighed over 300 pounds. This was probably the first recorded systematic application of progressive resistance to strength development.

Weightlifting competition with crude barbells and dumbbells began to develop in Europe in the mid-1500's, with Germany and France the chief centers of activity. Germany and France continued to be the main centers until 1896, when weightlifting was included as one of the events in the Modern Olympic Games. Most of the participants were heavy, big-boned men who had natural strength. It is doubtful that these men trained according to any kind of system.

Some interest in weight training began to develop in the United States during the closing years of the nineteenth century. Most of the interest was a result of the traveling strongman who toured the country and enthusiastically demonstrated lifting and muscle control. It was not until the early part of the twentieth century, however, that practical plateloading barbells and dumbbells were manufactured in the United States.

Although weight training became more widespread in the 1920's and 1930's, many misconceptions were generated during that period. Most of these beliefs were a result of faulty assumptions that weight lifting would make one slow and muscle bound, or would injure the heart. Interest in weight training reached a plateau as a result of these misconceptions, and then began to decline until World War II. During the war, many soldiers in Armed Forces training camps and hospitals personally experienced the benefits of the weight training. These men continued to train with weights after the war was over.

The popularity of weight training within the United States has been increasing since World War II. Today, millions of men exercise on a regular basis with the development of muscular size and strength as their primary goal.

The basic principles of body shaping and strength training for women apply equally well to men. Men, since they are usually stronger than women, will need more resistance to tax fully their muscles. Barbells and dumbbells are more practical for men to train with than cans and water-filled bottles.

Men should perform one set of 12 exercises, three times per week. A weight should be selected that allows the muscles to become exhausted between 8 to 12 repetitions. Particular emphasis should be placed on the lowering or negative phase of all exercises. The weight should always be smoothly raised and slowly lowered.

An example of a typical workout for a man is as follows:
1. Barbell squat
2. Back hyperextension
3. Chair step-up with dumbbell
4. Seated overhead press with barbell
5. Straight-armed pullover with barbell
6. Standing chair dip
7. Bent-over row with barbell
8. Triceps extension with one dumbbell

SPECIAL CONSIDERATIONS

9. Biceps curl with barbell
10. Neck exercises against arm resistance
11. Trunk curl
12. Reverse trunk curl

EXERCISE:
STRAIGHT-ARMED
PULLOVER WITH
BARBELL

RATING: A
EQUIPMENT:
BARBELL AND BENCH

Starting Position: Lie face-up on a bench. The head should be extended over the end. Hold the barbell over the chest in a straight-armed position.

Movement: Take a deep breath, lower the barbell behind the head, and return to the over-the-chest position. It is important to keep the arms straight during the movement and to emphasize the stretching of the torso when the barbell is behind the head. Repeat.

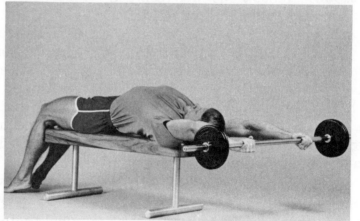

1

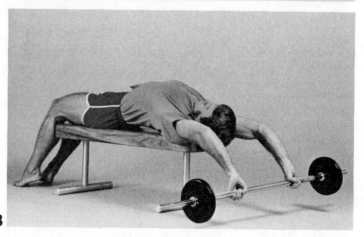

2

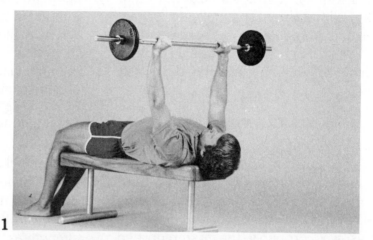

3

EXERCISE:
BARBELL SQUAT

RATING: A
EQUIPMENT:
BARBELL

Starting Position: Stand erect, feet shoulder-width apart, with a barbell secured in the hands and balanced across the shoulders. The feet should be flat if working the back is desired. The heels should be elevated if working the calves is preferable.

Movement: Slowly lower the upper body by bending the knees and hips. Look straight ahead or slightly upward during the movement. Continue downward until the thighs come into contact with the backs of the calves. **Do not** relax or bounce at the bottom of the movement. Return smoothly to the starting position and repeat.

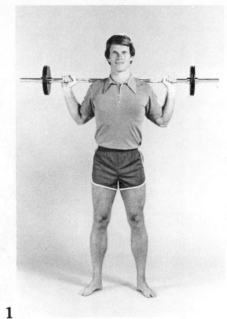

1

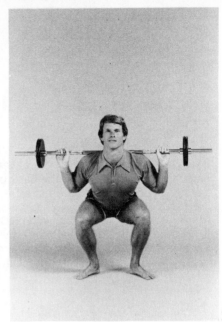

2

EXERCISE:
STANDING CHAIR DIP

RATING A
EQUIPMENT:
TWO CHAIRS

Starting Position: Face two chairs away from each other. Stand between them. Support the body on straightened arms against the backs of the chairs. Bend the legs at the knees.

Movement: Slowly lower the body by bending the arms. Stretch in the lower position and smoothly return to the top. Repeat.

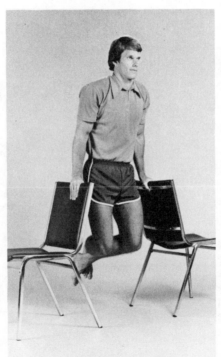

1

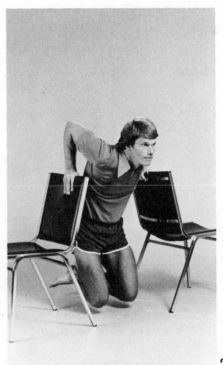

2

SPECIAL CONSIDERATIONS: MEN

EXERCISE:
REAR NECK EXTENSION AGAINST HAND RESISTANCE

RATING: A

EQUIPMENT: NONE

Starting Position: Interlace the fingers and place them on the back of the head. Chin should be on chest.

Movement: Push head back and resist the movement by pulling with the arms. Then pull forward with the arms and resist with the neck muscles. Repeat.

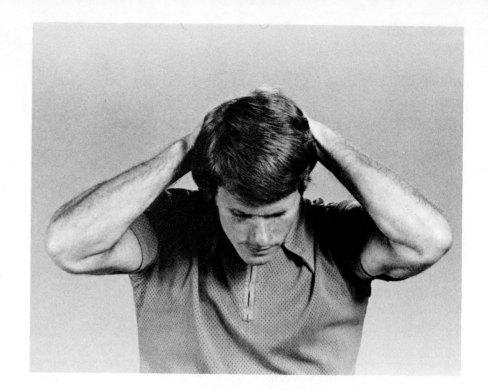

EXERCISE:
NECK FLEXION TO THE SIDE AGAINST HAND RESISTANCE

RATING: A

EQUIPMENT: NONE

Starting Position: With the head resting on the right shoulder, place the right hand just above the right ear.

Movement: Push the head to the left as far as it will go while resisting with the neck. Then use the neck to push the arm back to the starting position while resisting with the arm. After the right side of the neck is fatigued, reverse the procedure and work the left side of the neck against the left arm.

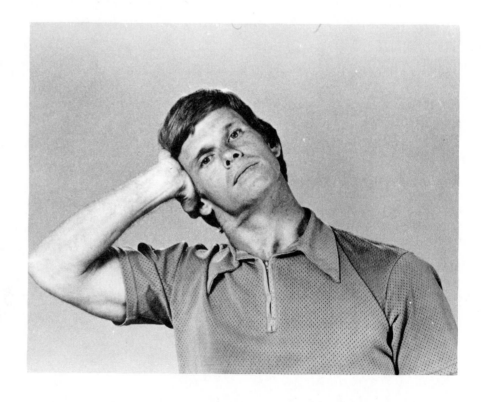

176

EXERCISE:
CHAIR STEP-UP WITH DUMBBELL

RATING: A
EQUIPMENT:
ONE CHAIR AND
ONE DUMBBELL

Starting Position: Stand erect with the left foot planted firmly in a straight-bottomed chair and the other foot on the floor. The dumbbell is held in one hand.

Movement: Slowly step up on the chair, then step down with the same leg and up again until it is completely fatigued. Switch sides and step up with the other leg.

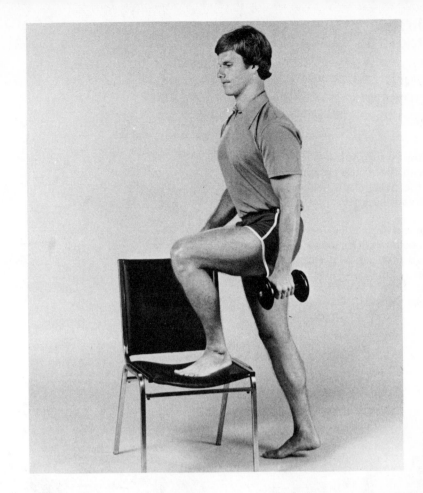

EXERCISE:
TRICEPS EXTENSION WITH ONE DUMBBELL

RATING: A
EQUIPMENT:
ONE DUMBBELL AND
BENCH

Starting Position: In a seated position, grasp a dumbbell in the left hand and raise it overhead. Keep the elbow by the ear.

Movement: Slowly bend and straighten the left arm. Do not move the elbows. Repeat. Follow the same directions for the right arm.

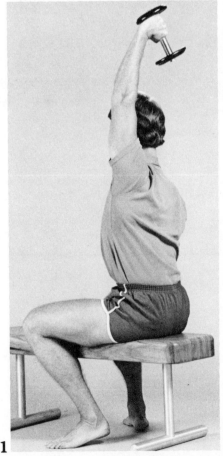

1

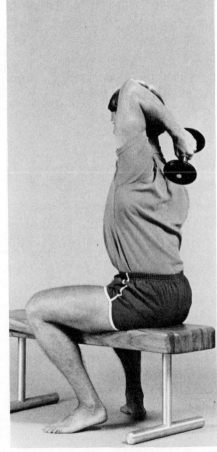

2

SPECIAL CONSIDERATIONS: MEN

EXERCISE:
TRUNK CURL

RATING: A
EQUIPMENT:
NONE

Starting Position: Lie face-up on the floor with the hands behind the head. Bring the heels close to the buttocks and spread the knees.

Movement: Try to curl the trunk to a sitting position. Only one third of a standard situp can be performed in this fashion. Pause in the contracted position. Slowly lower the trunk to the floor and repeat.

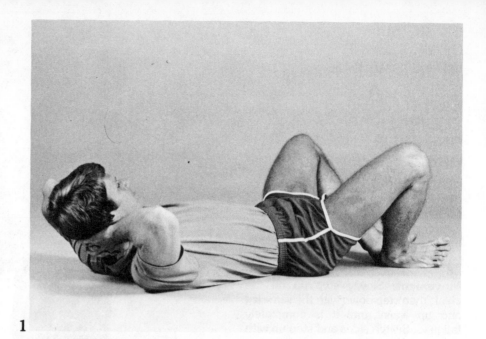

1

2

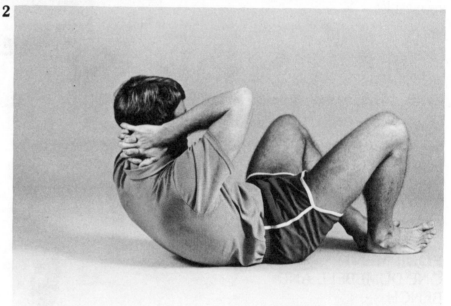

EXERCISE:
REVERSE TRUNK CURL

RATING A
EQUIPMENT:
NONE

Starting Position: Lie face-up on the floor with the hands on either side of the buttocks. Bring the thighs on the chest so the knees and hips are in a flexed position.

Movement: Curl the pelvic area toward the chin by lifting the buttocks and lower back. Pause. Slowly lower the buttocks and repeat.

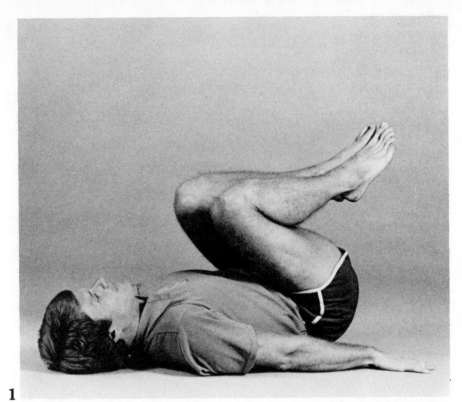

1

2

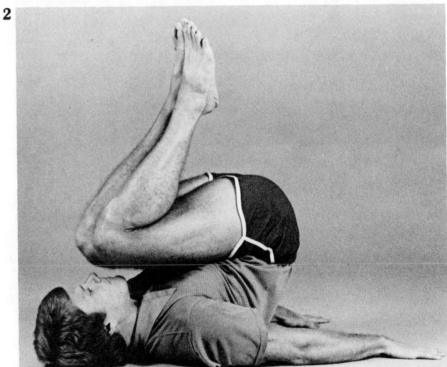

SPECIAL CONSIDERATIONS: MEN

EXERCISE:
BICEPS CURL
WITH BARBELL

RATING: A
EQUIPMENT:
BARBELL

Starting Position: Grasp a barbell with the palms up. Stand erect.

Movement: While keeping the body straight, smoothly curl the barbell. Slowly lower and repeat.

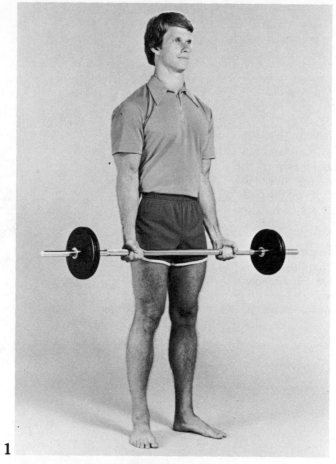

1

2

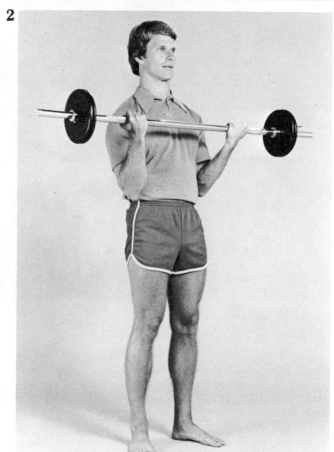

EXERCISE:
OVERHEAD PRESS
WITH BARBELL

RATING: B
EQUIPMENT:
BARBELL AND BENCH

Starting Position: Lift a barbell to the shoulders and sit on the end of a bench.

Movement: Press the barbell overhead and lower slowly back to shoulders. Repeat.

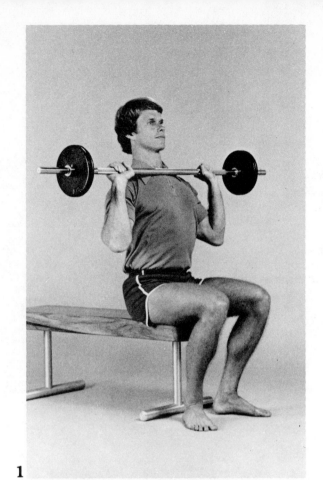

1

2

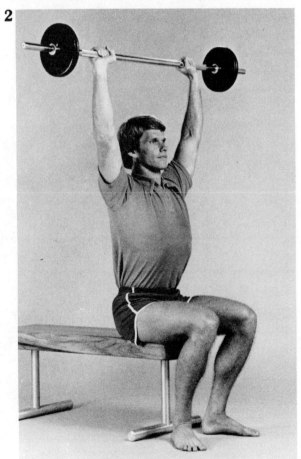

SPECIAL CONSIDERATIONS: MEN

EXERCISE:
BENT-OVER ROW WITH BARBELL

RATING: B
EQUIPMENT:
BARBELL

Starting Position: In a bent-over position, grasp a barbell with a narrow grip. The torso should be parallel with the floor.

Movement: Pull the hands upward until they touch the midsection. Pause. Slowly return to the starting position and repeat.

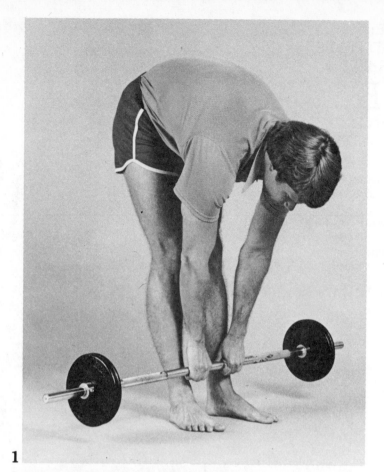

1

2

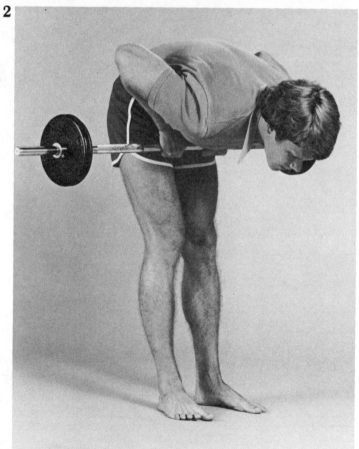

EXERCISE:
BACK HYPEREXTENSION

RATING: C
EQUIPMENT:
NONE

Starting Position: Lie face-down on the floor with entire body in a straight line. Interlace the hands behind the head.

Movement: Maintaining the legs firmly on the floor, attempt to raise the upper body slowly as high as possible off the floor. Pause. Lower and repeat.

1
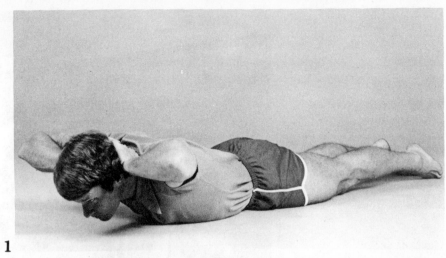

2
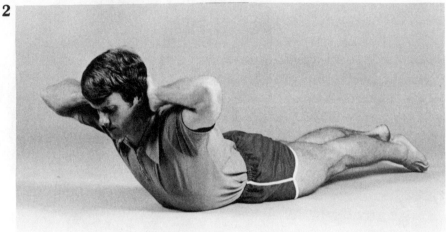

SPECIAL CONSIDERATIONS: MEN

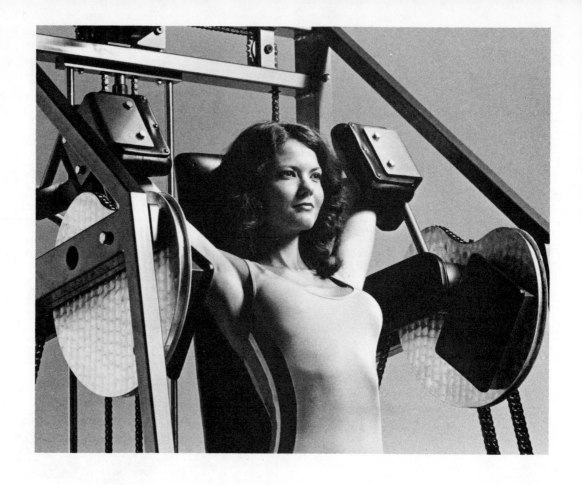

CHAPTER 17
ADVANCED BODY SHAPING

It usually takes from six months to a year of three-times-a-week, high-intensity exercise for a woman to be ready for advanced body shaping. After a year of steady training, most women will have doubled their strength in all major muscle groups. This is quite an accomplishment. It will significantly improve their performance in all sports and reduce the probability of many injuries. More importantly, her body from head to toe will be composed of firmer and shaplier flesh. But that should be just the first step. Her body-shaping and strengthening program can progress much higher.

Anyone considering an advanced body-shaping program must understand that the exercises are ranked in this book according to **the quantity of the movement by a specific part of the body and the quality of resistance applied against it.**

Exercises with short ranges of movement are not as productive as those with greater ranges. Exercises with moderate resistance are inferior to those with heavy or quality resistance. There are no easy ways to exercise. Even though it may be enjoyable, easy exercise produces very poor results.

Three simple but rigid rules must be applied for a woman to progress to an advanced body-shaping program:

1. Exercise **slower**.
2. Exercise **harder**.
3. Exercise **briefer**.

SLOWER

As a woman shapes and strengthens her body, she needs to pay closer and closer attention to the negative phase of each movement. For best results all negative movements must be performed slowly and smoothly. In the lowering portion of a pushup, the woman might picture herself in a slow-motion or stop-action movie. The film is projected frame-by-frame. She might imagine that she is the star of the show and as she descends the camera catches her -- click, one thousand and one; click, one thousand and two, and so on. The woman should time the movement so her body touches the floor at one thousand and four. Each of those "one thousands" equals one second. It is essential to remember that the negative portions of an exercise are most important for body shaping and strengthening. The woman should always perform them slowly and with great care.

HARDER AND BRIEFER

Advanced shaping and strenghtening of the feminine figure also requires a reduction of the total number of exercises. A woman's exercises must be reduced from 12 to 10, and her intensive training days from three days a week to two days a week. On Mondays and Fridays, she would still train at high intensity. The Wednesday program would be less strenuous. Each exercise would be stopped approximately two repetitions short of an all-out effort.

The Monday and Friday exercise sessions are the only ones that stimulate her body to get stronger. The Wednesday sessions simply prevent atrophy without depleting her valuable recovery ability.

BARBELLS AND DUMBBELLS

As a woman gets stronger, the resistance needed to produce the desired toning and shaping must increase. Plastic bottles filled with varying amounts of water will suffice up to a level of strength that requires no more than 10 pounds of resistance in each hand. Barbells and dumbbells offer an excellent means of progression past this level. In many respects, barbells and dumbbells are safer and easier to handle than household items. From 60 to 120 - pound sets of adjustable barbells and dumbbells are available at most sporting goods and department stores at a reasonable price. It would be a good investment for any figure-conscious woman.

NAUTILUS EQUIPMENT

One of the newest and most advanced body-shaping equipment is produced by Nautilus Sports/Medical Industries. Nautilus produces over 25 different exercise machines. There is a specific machine designed to shape the buttocks, the inner thighs, the chest, the waist, and all other major muscles. There are three machines for the neck alone. Any woman who lives close to a fitness center, university, or sports medicine clinic that has Nautilus machines, should use them.

The same body-shaping fundamentals explained in Chapter 2 apply to the use of Nautilus machines. A few of the most popular are pictured and described on the following pages.

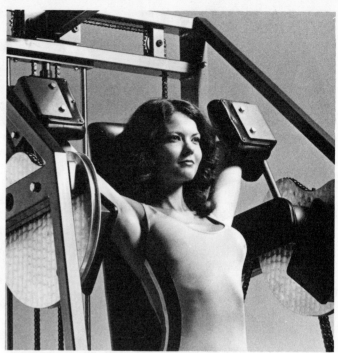

The Pullover-Torso machine exercises the strongest muscles of the upper body, the latissimus dorsi. The photograph shows the stretched starting position.

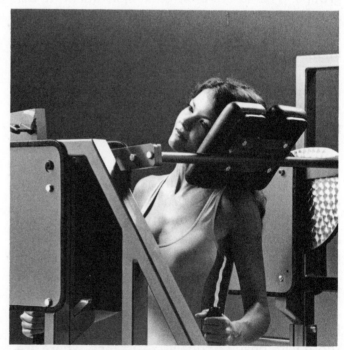

Women should not neglect the important muscles of the neck. Pictured above is lateral contraction of the neck to the left, one of four separate movements performed on the 4-Way Neck machine.

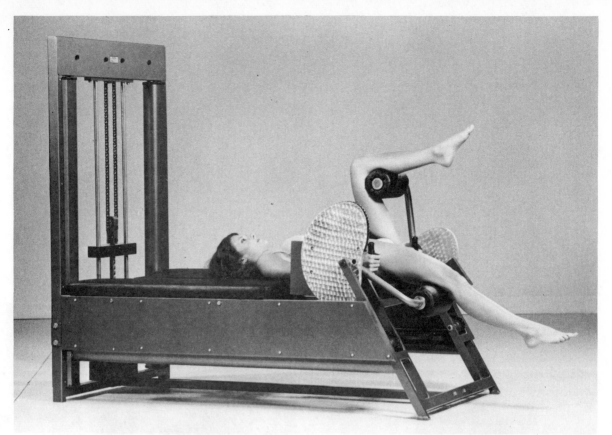

The largest yet most neglected muscles of the feminine figure are exercised directly on the Nautilus Hip and Back machine. Each buttock is alternately stretched and contracted throughout a full range of possible movement.

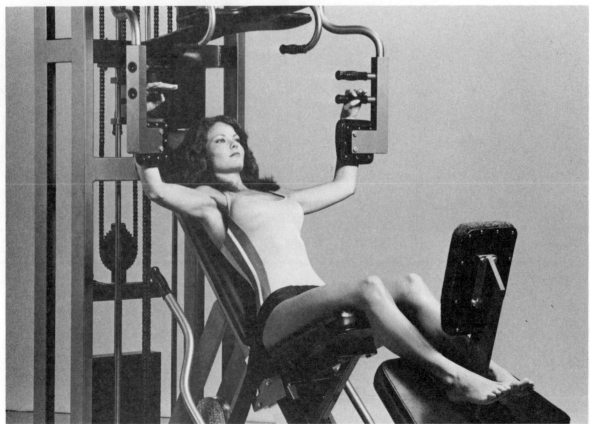

The function of the pectoralis major muscles of the chest is to move the upper arms across the front of the body. The arm cross on the Nautilus Double Chest machine allows the woman to effectively perform this movement against resistance.

SPECIAL CONSIDERATIONS: ADVANCED BODY SHAPING

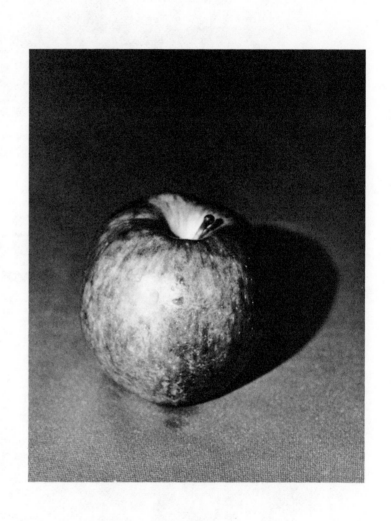

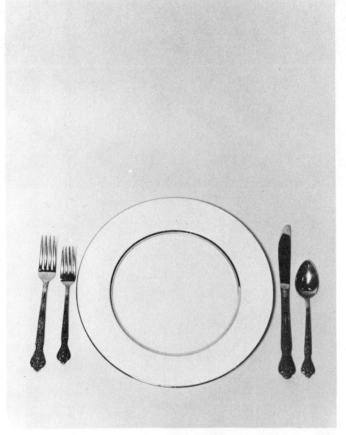

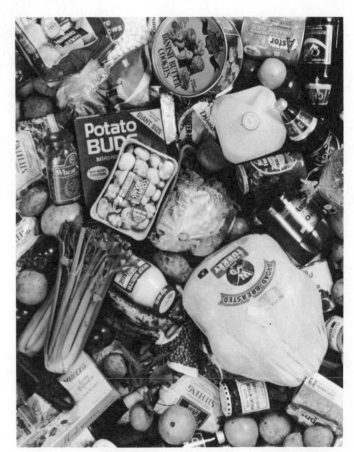

IV. DIET & NUTRITION

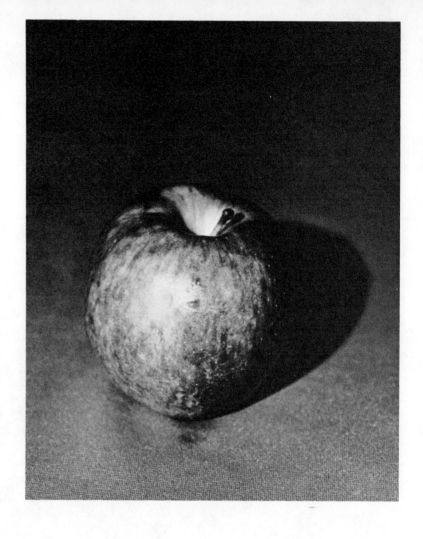

CHAPTER 18
THE BASICS OF NUTRITION

Life in the human organism is dependent upon an adequate dietary supply of nutrients: proteins, carbohydrates, fats, water, vitamins, and minerals. These nutrients occur in various combinations as foods. In order to meet our physiological need for these nutrients, we must eat a proper combination of different types of foods.

If all the solid food eaten during one day by an average woman were put in a half-gallon milk carton, the container would be about one-half full. If this mixture were transferred to a shallow dish and put in an oven at a temperature warm enough to evaporate the water without burning the food, the volume would be reduced eventually to less than a pint. Heating this residue in a laboratory oven at a much higher temperature would reduce the residue to about a level teaspoon.

This simple experiment tells much about the composition of food. A large percentage of the average American diet, excluding beverages, is water. Foods such as tomatoes, apples, and spinach contain over 85 percent water. Foods such as grains, flour, and cereal contain less than 15 percent water.

The pint of residue that remains after the water is evaporated comprises the carbohydrates, fats, proteins, vitamins, and minerals in this original sample of food. About one-half of the residue is carbohydrate, one-fourth protein, and one-fourth, fat. Vitamins and minerals represent a minute fraction of the total mixture. The teaspoon of ash remaining after the proteins, carbohydrates, fats and vitamins are burned off comprises the diet's minerals.

THE NUTRIENTS

Proteins, carbohydrates, fats, vitamins, and minerals are household words today. Their use is not limited to the biochemist, nutritionist, or dietician. These terms appear daily in newspaper columns, on food labels, and even in television advertisement for dog food and beer. Few people, however, know how a protein differs from a fat or a carbohydrate, or why large amounts of various vitamins and minerals are not necessary for vibrant health.

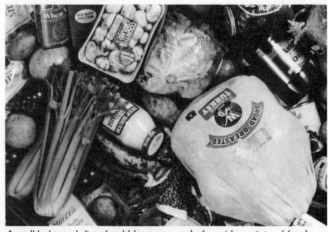

A well-balanced diet should be composed of a wide variety of food.

DIET AND NUTRITION

The following facts offer basic information for those women who want to know more about nutrition.

PROTEINS

All life requires protein. It is the chief tissue builder and the basic substance of every cell in the body.

Protein is made up of smaller units, called amino acids. After foods are eaten, the proteins are broken down -- digested -- into amino acids which are then rearranged to form the many special and distinct proteins in the body.

The proteins in food are usually made up of 18 or more amino acids. The body can make its own supply of more than half of these. But the others must come ready-made from food and are called essential amino acids.

The amino acid composition of a good protein determines its nutritive value. Proteins that supply all the essential amino acids in about the same proportions needed by the body are highest in value. Foods that provide large amounts of these top-ranking proteins meet the body's needs. Generally, these are foods of animal origin -- meat, fish, poultry, eggs, and milk.

Proteins from cereal grains, vegetables, and fruits provide fewer amino acids than animal proteins, but they do supply valuable amounts of many amino acids. Proteins from legumes, especially the soybeans, and chickpeas, are almost as good as proteins from animal sources.

For a woman's daily meals to rank well in protein quality, only a portion of the protein needs to come from animal sources. Combining cereal and vegetable foods with a little meat or other sources of animal protein will improve the protein value of the meal. Examples of nourishing combinations are cereal with milk, rice with fish, spaghetti with meat sauce, vegetable stew with meat. Or a person could simply have milk as a beverage along with foods of plant origin. It is good to have some food from animal sources at each meal.

Women need protein all through life for the maintenance and repair of body tissues. Children urgently need protein for normal growth.

Building of cells is only one of the roles of protein in the body. Protein performs the following functions:

- Makes hemoglobin, the blood protein that carries oxygen to the cells and carries carbon dioxide away from the cells.

- Forms antibodies that fight infection.

- Supplies energy if carbohydrates and fats are not available.

Adequate amounts of protein are found in meat, poultry, fish, milk, cheese, eggs, dry beans, dry peas, seeds, and nuts.

Bread, cereal, vegetables, and fruits contain relatively smaller amounts of protein. But the quantity of bread eaten daily may be large enough to make these foods important protein sources.

CARBOHYDRATES

Foods supply carbohydrates chiefly in three forms: starches, sugars, and cellulose or fibrous materials. Starches and sugars are major sources of energy for humans. Celluloses furnish bulk in the diet.

Glucose, commonly called blood sugar, is the form in which starches and sugars are mainly used by cells to furnish energy for body processes and to support activity and growth.

Carbohydrates spare proteins by supplying energy, thereby saving protein for tissue building and repair and for other special jobs. Carbohydrates also help the body use fats efficiently.

The chief sources of starch are grains such as wheat, oats, corn, and rice. Starches made from grains are flour, macaroni, spaghetti, noodles, grits, breads, and breakfast cereals. Potatoes, sweetpotatoes, and dry beans and peas are also sources of starch.

Most other vegetables, fruits, and fruit juices contain smaller amounts of carbohydrates. In vegetables this is mainly in the form of starches. In fruits it is chiefly sugars.

Cane and beet sugars, jellies, jam, candy and other sweets, honey, molasses, and syrups are concentrated sources of sugar.

FATS

Fats are concentrated sources of energy. Weight for weight, they give more than twice as much energy, or calories, as either carbohydrates or proteins.

Everyone needs some fat. Primarily the fats supply energy, but they also carry the fat-soluble vitamins A, D, E, and K.

Fats also perform the following functions:
• Make up part of the structure of cells
• Form a protective cushion around vital organs
• Spare protein for body building and repair by providing energy
• Supply an essential fatty acid, linoleic acid

The body does not manufacture linoleic acid so it must be provided by food. It is found in valuable amounts in many oils that come from plants -- particularly corn, cottonseed, safflower, sesame, soybean, and wheat grem. These are referred to as polyunsaturated fats or oils. Margarines, salad dressings, mayonnaise, and cooking oils are usually made from one or more of these oils. Nuts contain less linoleic acid than most vegetable oils. Among the nuts, walnuts rate quite high. Poultry and fish oils have more linoleic acid than other animal fats, which rank fairly low as sources.

In choosing daily meals, it is best to keep the total amount of fat at a moderate level and include some foods that contain polyunsaturated fats.

In cooking, fats add flavor and variety to many foods. Fats also make foods and meals satisfying because fats digest slowly and delay a feeling of hunger.

Common sources of fats are butter, margarine, shortening, cooking and salad oils, cream, most cheeses, mayonnaise, salad dressing, nuts, bacon, and other fatty meats. Meats, whole milk, eggs, and chocolate contain some fat naturally. Many popular snacks, baked goods, pastries, and other desserts are made with fat or cooked in it.

CHOLESTEROL

Cholesterol is a fat-like substance made in the body and found in every cell. It is a normal constituent of blood and tissues. In addition to the cholesterol made in the body, smaller amounts come from food. Cholesterol content of the diet is but one of many factors that influence the cholesterol level in blood.

Cholesterol is found only in foods of animal origin. It is not present in fruits, vegetables, cereal grains, legumes, or nuts, or in vegetable oils or other foods that come from plants. The highest concentrations of cholesterol are found in organ meats -- brain, liver, kidney, heart, sweetbreads, gizzards -- and in egg yolk. Shrimp is moderately high in cholesterol. Other foods of animal origin contain smaller amounts.

MINERAL ELEMENTS

Many minerals are required by the body. They give strength and rigidity to certain body tissues, and help with numerous vital functions.

CALCIUM

Calcium is the most abundant mineral element in the body. Teamed with phosphorus, it is largely responsible for the hardness of bones and teeth. About 99 percent of the calcium in the body is found in these two tissues.

The small amount of calcium in the body tissues and fluids aids in the proper functioning of the heart, muscles, and nerves, and helps the blood coagulate during bleeding.

Milk is outstanding as a source of calcium. Appreciable amounts are contributed by cheese, especially Cheddar types. Calcium is found in ice cream, collards, kale, mustard greens, turnip greens, and canned salmon.

DIET AND NUTRITION: THE BASICS OF NUTRITION

IODINE

People who live away from the seacoast in areas where the soil is low in iodine sometimes fail to get an adequate supply of this mineral. Getting too little iodine can cause goiter, a swelling of the thyroid gland.

Iodized salt and seafoods are reliable sources of iodine. Regular use of iodized salt is the most practical way to assure enough iodine in the diet.

IRON

Iron is needed by the body in relatively small but vital amounts. It combines with protein to make hemoglobin, which carries oxygen from the lungs to body cells and removes carbon dioxide from the cells. Iron also helps the cells obtain energy from food.

Only a few foods contain much iron. Liver is a particularly good source. Lean meats, heart, kidney, shellfish, dry beans, dry peas, dark-green vegetables, dried fruit, egg yolk, and molasses are also reliable sources.

Consumption of iron-rich foods is important for young children, pre-teen and teenage girls, and for women of childbearing age. Research shows these are the groups whose diets are most likely to be lacking in iron.

OTHER ESSENTIAL MINERALS

Two other minerals with vitally important functions are phosphorus and magnesium. Like calcium, they are found in largest amounts in bones and teeth. Among their other functions, they play an indispensable role in the body's use of food for energy.

Magnesium is found in adequate amounts in nuts, whole-grain products, dry beans, dry peas, and dark-green vegetables. Phosphorus is found in a variety of foods. If the meals contain foods that provide enough protein and calcium, a woman very likely will get enough phosphorus as well.

There are 10 or more essential minerals that help keep the body functioning in a smooth and orderly fashion. These minerals, however, will usually be provided in satisfactory amounts by a well-chosen variety of foods as outlined in the Daily Food Guide at the end of this chapter.

Fluoride, which helps protect teeth from decay, may be an exception. During the years when teeth are being formed, drinking water that contains a proper amount of fluoride, either natural or added, will make teeth more resistant to decay.

VITAMINS

Vitamins play a dynamic role in body processes. They take part in the release of energy from foods, promote normal growth of different kinds of tissue, and are essential to the proper functioning of nerves and muscle.

A dozen or more major vitamins that food must provide have been identified. Ordinarily, a woman can get all the vitamins she needs from a well-chosen assortment of everyday foods, such as is suggested in the Daily Food Guide.

Here is a summary of the vitamins, including some of the their functions and a list of foods that are dependable sources.

Vitamin A

Vitamin A occurs only in foods of animal origin. Many vegetables and fruits, however, particularly green and yellow ones, contain a substance called carotene that the body can change into vitamin A.

Liver is outstanding for vitamin A. Important amounts are also found in eggs, butter, margarine, whole milk, and cheese made with whole milk. Carotene is found in largest amounts in dark-green and deep-yellow vegetables and deep-yellow fruits.

Vitamin D

Vitamin D is important in building strong bones and teeth because it enables the body to use the calcium and phosphorus supplied by food.

Few foods contain much vitamin D naturally. Milk with vitamin D added is a practical source. Small amounts of vitamin D are present in egg yolks, butter, and liver. Larger amounts occur in sardines, salmon, herring, and tuna.

Another source is the vitamin D produced by action of direct sunlight on the skin.

To supplement amounts from sunlight and food, vitamin D preparations may be prescribed by a physician for infants and young children.

Ascorbic Acid (Vitamin C)

Ascorbic acid helps form and maintain cementing material that holds body cells together and strengthens the walls of blood vessels. It also assists in normal tooth and bone formation and aids in healing wounds.

Oranges, grapefruit, lemons, and fresh strawberries are rich in ascorbic acid. Other important sources include tomatoes, broccoli, cabbage, cantaloupe, cauliflower, green and red peppers, some dark-green leafy vegetables, and watermelon.

The B Vitamins

Three of the B vitamins—thiamin, riboflavin, and niacin—play a central role in the release of energy from food. They also help with proper functioning of nerves, normal appetite, good digestion, and healthy skin.

Body Use	Nutrient Group		Food Sources
Nutrients that produce energy (calories)	*Carbohydrates*	*Sugar* *Starch*	Sugar, starch, syrup, cereals, candy, honey, jam, jelly, fruits, vegetables, most desserts.
	Fats	*Saturated* *Unsaturated*	Butter, margarine, cream, lard, cooking oils, vegetable shortening, meat fat, olives, nuts, chocolate, peanut butter, ice cream, whole milk, cheese, avocados, pastries, many batters and doughs.
Nutrients that build or repair tissue	*Proteins*	*Complete* *Incomplete*	Eggs, meat, fish, poultry, milk, cheese, legumes, nuts, cereals, especially whole grain cereals.
	Minerals		Milk, cheese, meat, egg, fruits, vegetables, legumes, whole grain and enriched cereals.
	Water		Water, milk, beverages, broth, all foods containing varying amounts of water.
Nutrients that regulate and coordinate life processes	*Vitamins*	*Water-soluble* *Fat-soluble*	Milk, fruits, vegetables, meat, eggs, whole grain and enriched cereals.
	Fiber (cellulose)		Fruits, vegetables, whole grain cereals.

Foods in the meat group of the Daily Food Guide are leading sources of these vitamins. Whole-grain and enriched bread and cereals supply smaller but important amounts. A few foods are outstanding sources: milk for riboflavin, lean pork for thiamin, and organ meats for all three.

Getting enough niacin is not a problem if enough protein is included in daily meals. An essential amino acid, tryptophan, present in protein, can be changed by the body into niacin.

Other B vitamins, B6 and particularly B12 and folic acid, help prevent anemia. Vitamin B12 is found only in foods of animal origin. The other two are widely distributed in foods. Folic acid occurs in largest amounts in organ meats and dark-green leafy vegetables. Good sources of Vitamin B6 include meats, whole-grain cereals, dry beans, potatoes, and dark-green, leafy vegetables.

Other Vitamins

Combinations of food that provide sufficiently for the vitamins above are likely to furnish enough of the other vitamins not specified.

WATER

Water is essential for life. It ranks next to air, or oxygen, in importance. The body's need for water even exceeds its need for food. A person can live for days, even weeks, without food, but only a few days without water.

About one-half to two-thirds of the body is made up of water. Water is the medium of body fluids, secretions, and excretions. It carries food materials from one part of the body to the other.

Also, water is the solvent for all products of digestion. It holds them in solution and permits them to pass through the intestinal wall into the bloodstream for use throughout the body. Water also carries wastes from the body. Body temperature is regulated by the evaporation of water through the skin and lungs.

It takes a regular and generous intake of water to perform all these jobs. The body gets water from many sources. The most obvious is the water you drink, but this often represents only a small part of the total intake. Water also comes in coffee, tea, juice, soft drinks, milk, and soups. Foods, such as vegetables, fruits, meat, and even bread and dry cereals, contain some water. And water is formed when the body uses food for energy.

DAILY FOOD GUIDE

Active people need adequate amounts of proteins, fats, carbohydrates, vitamins, minerals, and water on a daily dasis. Nutrition scientists have translated knowledge of the nutrient needs of people and the nutrient values of food into an easy-to-use guide for food selection.

This Daily Food Guide sorts foods into four groups on the basis of their similarity in nutrient content. Each of the broad groups has a special contribution to make to an adequate diet.

Daily Food Guide

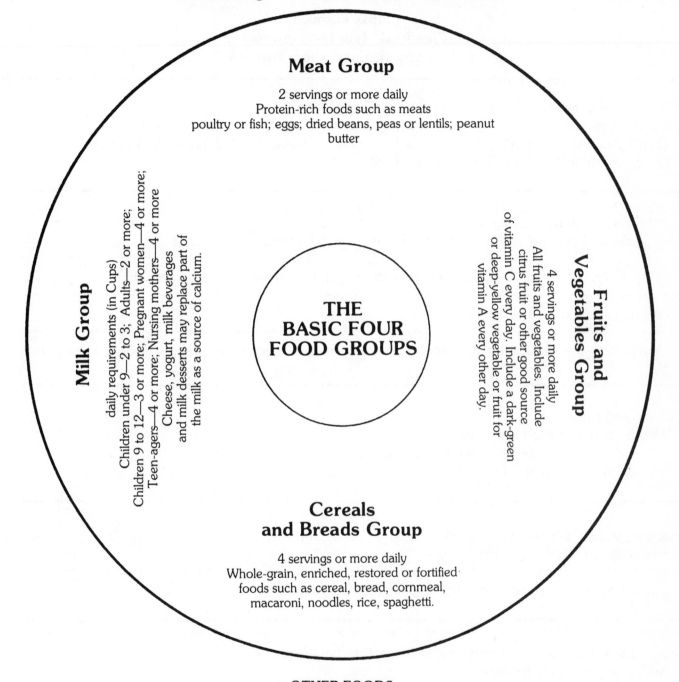

Meat Group

2 servings or more daily
Protein-rich foods such as meats
poultry or fish; eggs; dried beans, peas or lentils; peanut
butter

Milk Group

daily requirements (in Cups)
Children under 9—2 to 3; Adults—2 or more;
Children 9 to 12—3 or more; Pregnant women—4 or more;
Teen-agers—4 or more; Nursing mothers—4 or more
Cheese, yogurt, milk beverages
and milk desserts may replace part of
the milk as a source of calcium.

THE BASIC FOUR FOOD GROUPS

Fruits and Vegetables Group

4 servings or more daily
All fruits and vegetables. Include
citrus fruit or other good source
of vitamin C every day. Include a dark-green
or deep-yellow vegetable or fruit for
vitamin A every other day.

Cereals and Breads Group

4 servings or more daily
Whole-grain, enriched, restored or fortified
foods such as cereal, bread, cornmeal,
macaroni, noodles, rice, spaghetti.

OTHER FOODS

To add variety and additional calories, other foods not specified in the Basic
Four Food Groups may be used. Such foods include butter, margarine, oil, salad dressing, gravies, sauces,
sugars, jams, jellies, candies, syrups,
sweet desserts, sweetened and alcoholic beverages.

DIET AND NUTRITION: THE BASICS OF NUTRITION

Food Selection Scorecard

A woman should score her diet for each day using the points allowed for each food group. If her score is between 90 and 100, her food selection standard has been good; a score of 75 to 85 indicates a fair standard; a score below 75 is a low standard.

**Points allowed
(See basic four food groups
for serving size and substitutions.)**

Milk (include cheese, ice cream, and milk used in cooking)
    Adults: 1 glass, 10 points; 1½ glasses, 15; 2 glasses, 20.
    Teen-agers and children 9 to 12: 1 glass, 5 points; 2 glasses, 10; 3 glasses, 15; 4 glasses, 20.
    Children under 9: 2 glasses, 15; 3 glasses, 20.

Vegetables and fruits (serving = ½ cup)
    Vegetables: 1 serving, 5; 2 servings, 10. Potatoes may be included as one of these servings.

    Using 1 serving of a dark-green or deep-yellow vegetable will earn you 5 extra points.

    Fruits: 1 serving, 5; 2 servings, 10.

    Using citrus fruit, raw cabbage, canned or raw tomatoes, berries, or melons gives 5 extra points.

Cereals and breads
    Whole grain, enriched, or restored:
        Bread, rice, breakfast cereals, macaroni, etc.:
        2 servings, 10 points; 4 servings, 15.

Meat, eggs, fish, poultry, dried peas or beans, peanut butter:
    1 serving, 10; 2 servings, 15.

    Using 1 serving liver or other organs gives 5 extra points.

Total liquids (include milk, broth, tea, coffee, other beverages)
    Adults: 6 glasses, 3; 8 glasses, 5.
    Children: 4 glasses, 3; 6 glasses, 5.

Eating a breakfast which includes food from the meat or milk group. Do not count cream or bacon (except Canadian bacon) in the score.
10 points.

Maximum points for each group	Columns for daily check									
	1	2	3	4	5	6	7	8	9	10
20										
10										
5										
10										
5										
15										
15										
5										
5										
10										
100										

DIET AND NUTRITION: THE BASICS OF NUTRITION

Breakfast
Whole Orange
Brown rice with honey and milk
Mixed grain toast with margarine
Lightly toasted cashew nuts
Cereal coffee with low-fat milk

Lunch
Baked soybeans
Parslied potatoes
Carrot strips
Tossed green salad
    with sliced hard
    cooked eggs
Herb oil dressing
Rye bread with
    margarine
Pineapple juice

Dinner
Corn chowder
Whole wheat toast
    with apple butter
Small banana
Non-fat milk

CHAPTER 19
POPULAR REDUCING DIETS

The words weight and fat are frequently used in discussing the human body. Yet these terms are often misunderstood.

Body weight is simply what a person's entire body weighs. This is usually measured on pressure - or balance - type scales and is recorded in pounds or kilograms. The two major components of body weight, and certainly the most changeable, are muscle and fat.

Body fat is composed of three types of fat: subcutaneous, depot, and essential. A woman's body fat cannot be measured as accurately as her body weight.

Overweight is a term that in recent years has been determined by referring to the popular height-weight charts. Most of these charts have descended from averages of men and women who had bought life insurance policies between 1885 and 1908. Even though they have been updated, many questions still arise as to their accuracy. What about the variance of a woman's body weight depending on the time of day, season clothing, and state of digestion? Or what about her body build? Does she have a large, medium or small frame? If she has wide hips, how does she know if the extra width is from bone or fat? And what about her ethnic background? The concept of overweight may lead to more misconceptions then understanding.

Over fat is an idea can be understood by most people. Over fat is a bodily condition marked by excessive deposition and storage of fat. The key word is fat! It is not unusual to see women who are within the desirable ranges of the height-weight charts and are still over fat. Or they can be overweight and not over fat, or underweight, and actually over fat. It all depends on the amount of muscle and the amount of fat that a woman has on her body.

Fitness-minded women will function more efficiently with less fat and more muscle. Muscle gives the body shape, tone, and firmness. While some fat contributes to the feminine shape, most of it does the opposite. It contributes to a loose, flabby, unfashionable appearance.

A chemical analysis of a pound of muscle and a pound of fat reveals the following:

	Calories	Water	Lipids	Proteins
Muscle	600	70%	7%	22%
Fat	3,500	22%	72%	6%

The density of muscle is much greater than that of fat. Muscle is mostly water. Fat is mostly lipids, a greasy waxy substance. A pound of fat floats in water, while muscle sinks.

It is important to understand the physiological

DIET AND NUTRITION

facts that distinguish between muscle and fat. Most popular reducing diets make little distinction between these two factors.

Many diets are successful temporarily because they produce rapid weight loss. It is physically impossible to lose fat quickly. Weight quickly -- yes! Fat quickly -- no!

Weight lost quickly usually comes from the muscles, vital organs, and extra cellular fluid because they are composed primarily of water. A gallon of water weighs 8 pounds and some women can lose that much over a weekend. Losing water from the body, however, is not healthy. It upsets the body's delicate chemical balance and can lead to severe complications.

Unusual diets that differ significantly in composition from what the dieter is accustomed to eating will cause a temporary imbalance of fluids. This will not lead to a permanent loss of fat or weight.

CHERYL AND THE SCALES HOW NOT TO LOSE 5 POUNDS IN A DAY

Cheryl is a 30-year-old housewife with two children. She is happily married but has one annoying problem. She is getting fat and out of shape.

When the scales registered 140 pounds, she made up her mind to do something about that fat. She had not played tennis in several years. Acting on the determination to lose that fat, she went to the tennis court and played for three hours in the broiling sun. She skipped lunch and took a sauna bath until she almost dropped from exhaustion.

Staggering out of the sauna bath, she got on the scales. To her delight she had lost five pounds.

That evening, she had guests for dinner. With the cocktails, the trout amandine, all the extra dishes, and a rich dessert, Cheryl's dinner was high in both calories and fluid. When her guests left, she got on the scales. To her horror, the scales read, not 135, not 140, but 142 pounds.

What happened to the five pounds Cheryl had lost that afternoon?

Weak after the sauna, she had drunk two glasses of water. At home, she drank a large ginger ale while helping the maid prepare dinner for her guests. Before dinner, she joined her friends in several cocktails. Along with the four-course meal she drank two glasses of wine and another glass of water. Her total food and drink intake was approximately 112 ounces, or seven pounds.

At the tennis court and in the sauna, Cheryl had lost five pounds of water from sweat. None of this water came from her stored fat. All the liquid she had drunk along with the food at the dinner party not only replaced but increased the fluid she had lost on the tennis court and in the sauna.

Cheryl intended to lose fat, but all she lost was weight in the form of sweat. The total number of calories she consumed for the day was 2,650. Her total caloric expenditure was 2,550. She came out with 100 surplus calories and added 1/35 of a pound to her other fat.

One pint of water weighs one pound. A gallon of water weighs 8 pounds. An over fat woman can lose 4 or 5 pounds from sweat on a hot afternoon or in a sauna bath. Fluid loss has to be replaced. Nature forces the body through thirst to return to its fluid equilibrium.

There is only one way to lose fat: Expend more calories than are consumed. Fat loss and weight loss are two different processes. Weight can be lost quickly. Fat cannot.

Even diets that produce fat loss slowly will most likely cause some loss of water from the muscles. This can be prevented if the dieter trains her body in a high-intensity exercise program several times a week. High-intensity exercise makes the muscles stronger and shaplier. The goals of a woman who wants to reduce her bodyweight should be as follows:

1. To lose fat safely
2. To lose fat slowly
3. To lose fat permanently
4. To stimulate muscles to become stronger and shaplier.

Some popular diets adhere to these four principles of reducing body weight. Other diets ignore the principles.

LOW-CARBOHYDRATE DIETS

Low-carbohydrate diets are those that reduce the amount of carbohydrates a person eats at each meal. The dieter maintains the same amount, or slightly lower amount, of fats and proteins that she ate before beginning the diet. Although there are numerous variations of this diet, the general agreement seems to be that the dieter's carbohydrate intake should not exceed 60 grams a day. Nor should it fall below 50 grams.

An example of a typical low-carbohydrate diet for one day is as follows:

Breakfast
    1 cup strawberries
    1 egg
    1 slice bread with 1 tsp. cream cheese
    1 cup skim milk
    coffee or tea as desired

Lunch
    4 ounces tuna fish
    1 slice bread
    ½ cup skim milk
    1 small banana

Dinner
    ½ cup green peas
    1 slice bread
    2 ounces chicken breast
    ½ cup skim milk
    coffee or tea as desired

HIGH-PROTEIN DIETS

High-protein diets emphasize protein foods and limit carbohydrates and fats. These diets are based primarily on the belief that higher protein consumption requires more calorie use in digestion and metabolism. Protein foods do require slightly more dynamic action in the body than a balanced diet. Perhaps two percent more calories are burned by the protein.

Some of the high-protein diets allow people to eat all they want of certain foods, such as lean meats and poultry, fish and seafood, and eggs. Most people, however, soon get tired of consuming large amounts of those foods. They actually do eat less food than they have been eating.

The following is an example of a high-protein diet:

Breakfast
    2 ounces orange juice
    1 egg
    1 piece melba toast

Lunch
    4 ounces lean meat or fish
    1 piece of melba toast
    1 cup salad with low-calorie dressing
    1 apple
    ½ cup gelatin dessert

Dinner
    5 ounces of meat or fish
    1 piece of melba toast
    1 cooked vegetable
    1 cup salad with low-calorie dressing
    ½ cup gelatin dessert

To Drink At Any Time
Coffee, tea, diet soda, tomato juice, skim milk

HIGH-FAT DIETS

Many diets that are high in protein are also high in fat. A gram of protein has 4 calories and a gram of fat has 9 calories. Three ounces of broiled round steak, for example, contains 215 calories: 98 calories from protein and 117 from fat. Again carbohydrate foods are avoided on such a diet.

High-fat menus include an abundance of such dishes as chicken salad with mayonnaise, seafood with lemon butter sauce, cheese omelet with bacon, and eggs Benedict with hollandaise sauce. No fruits, vegetables, sugars, starches, breads, ice cream or other foods with carbohydrates can be included in high-fat menus.

THE LIQUID DIET

For some people the epitome of pleasure is associated with sitting down to a meal, consuming crunchy and juicy food and appreciating the sensual textures of mastication. They appreciate food so much, in fact, they often eat too much of it. One of the answers for them may be the liquid diet.

Basically, there are two types of liquid diets: the nutritionally milk-based 900-calorie formulas, and the predigested protein sirups which can be mixed with water and substituted for all other foods.

The 900-calorie formulas are milk based and include corn or coconut oils, soy flour, and added vitamins and minerals. In the simplest version they come in cans. Each 10-ounce can consists of 225 calories, four cans making up the day's meals. One can contains approximately 11 grams of protein, 35 grams of carbohydrates, and 5 grams of fat.

The pre-digested protein mixture is lacking in two of the usual nutrients: fats and carbohydrates. Heavily flavored with artificial sweetener, it is totally extracted from beef hides. Two tablespoons contains 60 calories and 15 grams of protein, no fats and no carbohydrates. A daily intake of four to seven ounces will provide the dieter with 300 to 500 calories.

Liquid dieting is not a normal or long-term way of eating. Many people feel deprived of the pleasures of sharing a meal at the table. Others suffer negative effects such as constipation, diarrhea, dizziness, dry skin, hair loss, nausea, gas and bad breath.

A liquid diet should only be followed under a physician's guidance.

MINI-CALORIE DIETS

The ultimate mini-calorie diet is fasting. This is the easiest and cheapest diet of all because the individual does not count calories, carbohydrates or anything except the two quarts of water she must drink every day. Over fat people can survive for a long time without food, but without water they would be dead in few days. Most weight-reducing fasts last less than a week.

Some people, rather than totally fast, choose what is called a modified fast. A modified fast often entails fruit and vegetable juices. These fasters supplement their water drinking with varying amounts of orange, lemon, tomato, carrot, grapefruit, and any other kinds of juices. Other fasters drink cups of hot beef or chicken bouillon or clear vegetable broth.

Breaking the fast is the most important part of the program. It is essential not to overload the system following a fast. Perhaps here is the opportune time for the person to retrain herself into nutritionally sound eating habits. The idea is to increase the amount of food gradually.

There are two unbreakable rules of fasting:

First, the person should consult a physician before beginning a fast of more than a day or two. Some people should never fast, those with heart or liver disease, for example.

Second, the faster should start eating again when true hunger returns. With the return of physiological hunger, the woman's body is warning her that it has used up most of her stored nourishment. To keep alive the body must now increase mobilization of essential protein tissues, a deadly dangerous prospect.

VEGETARIAN DIETS

There are several classifications of vegetarian diets:

1. **Strict vegetarian:** Only foods of plant origin, including seeds, nuts, fruits and vegetables.

2. **Lacto-vegetarian:** All foods of plant origin, plus foods made of milk.

3. **Lacto-ovo-vegetarian:** All foods of plant origin, plus foods made of milk, plus eggs.

Nutritionists are in agreement that a vegetarian diet can be safe as long as it provides some protein from dairy products or from fish or eggs. A diet heavy in vegetables and fruits will still lack some B vitamins, especially B12.

SAMPLE VEGETARIAN DIETS

Lacto-ovo-vegetarian

Breakfast
  Whole orange
  Brown rice with honey and milk
  Mixed grain toast with margarine
  Lightly toasted cashew nuts
  Cereal coffee with low-fat milk

Lunch
  Baked soybeans
  Parslied potatoes
  Carrot strips
  Tossed green salad
    with sliced hard
    cooked eggs
  Herb oil dressing
  Rye bread with
    margarine
  Pineapple juice

Dinner
  Corn chowder
  Whole wheat toast
    with apple butter
  Small banana
  Non-fat milk

Strict Vegetarian

Breakfast
  Whole orange
  Brown rice with
    honey and soy milk
  Mixed grain toast
    with margarine
  Lightly toasted cashew
    nuts
  Cereal coffee with
    soy milk

Lunch
  Baked soybeans
  Parslied potatoes
  Carrot strips
  Tossed green salad
    with garbanzos
  Herb oil dressing
  Rye bread with
    margarine
  Pineapple juice

Dinner
  Corn chowder made
    with soy milk
  Whole wheat toast
    with apple butter
  Small banana
  Soy milk

THE SINGLE-FOOD DIETS

Many dieters, who find monotony no problem, may consider a single-food diet. Such foods as grapefruit, bananas, tomatoes, eggs, and yogurt head the list of one-food regimes. Actually, the diets include other foods, but they do center on several servings a day of a single food.

A typical example is the Grapefruit Diet:

Breakfast
  ½ grapefruit or
    unsweetened grapefruit
    juice
  2 eggs, any style
  Minimum 2 slices of bacon --
    more if desired
  Coffee or tea, no sugar

Lunch
  ½ grapefruit
  Meat, any style, any amount
  Salad, any amount, with
    any dressing that
    contains no sugar
  Coffee or tea

Dinner
  ½ grapefruit
  Meat, any style, any
    amount, or fish
  Green, yellow or red

vegetable in any
amount
Salad as above
Coffee or tea

Bedtime Snack
Tomato juice or
skim milk

The Grapefruit Diet is sold on the premise that grapefruit has certain enzymes that somehow subtract calories, by acting as a catalyst to increase the fatburning process. This concept is disclaimed by nutritionists, who insist that while grapefruit is a nutritious food, it has no magic power to burn away fat.

LOW-CALORIE DIETS

All food and drink, with the exception of water, coffee, tea, and diet sodas, contain calories in varying amounts. From a single bite of raw celery to the stickiest fudge sundae ever created, there are calories to count and contend with. The body uses calories as fuel, burning off 3,500 calories to lose one pound of fat. Each food, by a specified number, has a caloric count. The calorie count is the heat energy that a particular food can yield as it passes through the body.

To lose fat by counting calories, a woman would have to first find out how many calories it takes merely to maintain her normal weight. A moderately active 5 foot 7 inch woman needs about 2,240 calories a day.

For this woman to lose a pound of fat, she will have to cut out 3,500 calories from her weekly intake. She must eat 500 fewer calories from her daily intake. She must eat 500 fewer calories per day, or a total of 1,640. For a two-pound loss per week, her calories must be reduced by 1,000 per day to 1,240.

The following is an example of well-balanced, low-calorie meals for one day.

1,000 CALORIE MENU

Breakfast, 205 calories
½ cup fresh diced pineapple
1 slice honey ham loaf
1 slice low-calorie toast
1 teaspoon low-calorie margarine
¼ cup cottage cheese
Coffee or tea

Lunch, 385 calories
3-½ ounces tuna fish
½ cauliflower, boiled or raw
1 slice low-calorie bread
1 banana
½ cup skim milk
Coffee or tea

Dinner, 410 calories
4 ounces lean roast beef
1 baked potato without skin
1 tablespoon sour cream
1 slice low-calorie bread
½ cup strawberries
Diet soda

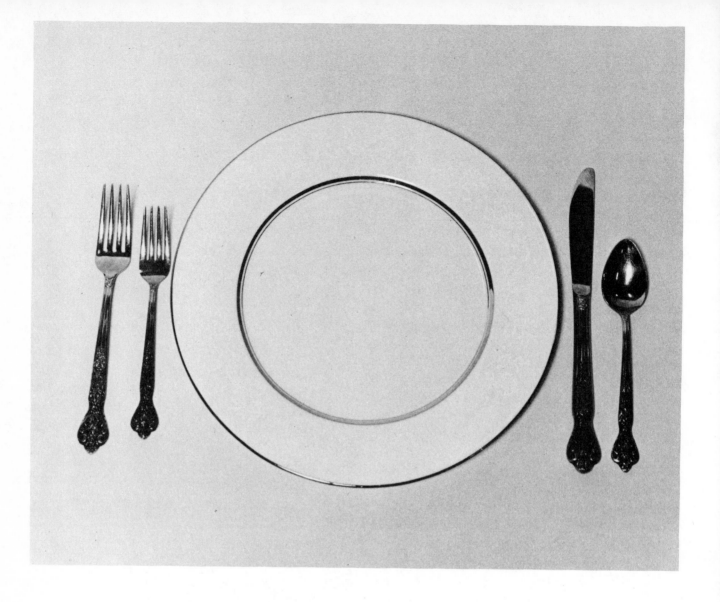

CHAPTER 20
HOW TO CHOOSE A DIET

Americans display an almost undiscriminating love of food. Fast food, health food, high-protein, high-fat, low-carbohydrate, low-calorie, ethnic dishes, soul food, and good old American apple pie a la mode—we love it all. Family and social life centers on food. A full stomach means that, for the moment at least, all is well.

But all is not well within the bodies of most Americans. For these bodies have been misshapen by fat, sagging muscles, clogged arteries, and other ills. But the fat and flaccid shape and condition of Americans can be changed. This change can be effected by understanding and applying **Consumer Guide's** rules for evaluating dietary programs.

1. Beware of a diet on which an author or publisher is making money from the sales of special supplies and supplements.
2. Consider a diet experimental until it has ample evidence of its effectiveness from recognized scientific research which has been published in reputable medical journals.
3. Ignore diets based on some "secret" formula. There is no secret formula for losing fat.
4. Accept a low-calorie diet only if it is well-balanced. Diets heavy in protein and fat or low in carbohydrates are not balanced. Diets lower than 1,000 calories a day can be dangerous.
5. Be cautious of a diet offered by anyone who does not have an earned degree in nutrition from an accredited university.

NUTRITIONAL REQUIREMENTS FOR A BALANCED DIET

The important factor in losing body fat is the strict adherence to a diet restricted in calories but balanced in nutrients.

The foods necessary to supply all the nutrients for the repair, growth, and energy needs of the body can be divided into four basic groups:
1. Meat
2. Dairy products
3. Fruits and vegetables
4. Breads and cereals

Besides the four basic food groups, there are foods such as candy, soft drinks, butter, margarine, salad dressings, and certain snacks that contribute little except calories to the diet.

MEAT GROUP
The meat group is composed of meat, fish, cheese, beans, dry peas, eggs, nuts, and poultry. These foods are all high in protein and ample amounts of fat. Daily intake should include two or more servings, preferably with each meal supplying some protein from these sources.

DAIRY PRODUCTS
Adults do not outgrow their need for dairy products. At least two servings a day are needed. This group includes whole and skimmed milk, buttermilk, yogurt, cheese, cottage cheese, and

DIET AND NUTRITION

ice cream. Protein, fat, and calcium are all found in dairy products.

FRUITS AND VEGETABLES

Servings of fruit and vegetables should amount to three or four a day including both green and yellow varieties. Fruits and vegetables are excellent sources of carbohydrates, vitamins, and minerals.

BREADS AND CEREALS

Breads and cereals include enriched or whole-grain products. Three or four servings should be eaten every day. Though the primary contribution of this group is carbohydrate energy, it also contains protein, vitamins, and minerals.

OTHER FOODS

All foods in this group are primarily sources of energy; some, like butter or margarine, contribute vitamin A. By themselves, they cannot nourish and sustain the body, but they do add flavor and variety to meals, satisfy appetites, and add to the joy of living.

There is danger, however, that these extras may crowd out important food. When fat must be reduced, this group of foods is the first and best place to eliminate.

The following chart, based on selections from the four basic food groups, should be useful to all dieters. This chart furnishes guidelines for diets of 1,200 and 1,500 calories.

DIETARY GUIDELINES FOR LOSING FAT

FOOD	FOR 1,200 CALORIES DAILY	FOR 1,500 CALORIES DAILY	NOTES
Meat Group	3 small servings (or a total of 7 ounces cooked weight)	3 small servings (or a total of 7 ounces cooked weight)	Choose lean, well-trimmed meats: beef, veal, lamb, pork. Poultry and fish should have skin removed. One egg can be substituted for 1 serving of meat.
Dairy Products	2 cups fortified skim milk	2 cups whole milk	Two cups milk means two 8-ounce measuring cups.
Fruits and Vegetables	4 servings	4 servings	One fruit serving = 1 medium fruit, 2 small fruits, ½ banana, ¼ cantaloupe, 10-12 grapes or cherries, 1 cup fresh berries or ½ cup fresh, canned or frozen unsweetened fruit or fruit juice. Include one citrus fruit or other good source of vitamin C daily. One vegetable serving = ½ cup cooked or 1 cup raw leafy vegetable. Include one dark green or deep yellow vegetable or other good source of vitamin A at least every other day.
	NOTE: Because of space limitations, calorie tables are not included in this book. There are many inexpensive, paperback books that provide this information.		
Breads and Cereals	4 servings	5 servings	One serving = 1 slice bread; 1 small dinner roll; ½ cup cooked cereal, noodles, macaroni, spaghetti, rice, cornmeal; 1 ounce (about 1 cup) ready to eat unsweetened iron-fortified cereal.
Other Foods	1 serving	3 servings	One serving = 1 teapoon butter, margarine, or oil; 6 nuts; 2 teaspoons salad dressing; or 35 calories or less of another food.

TRICKS THAT
CONTROL HUNGER

Three physiological subsystems are involved in hunger: the brain, the gut, and the endocrine system. These subsystems are subject to mental, physical, and social control.

The first line of defense against the appetite is the hypothalamus. The hypothalamus is the control center of the brain. Signals that dieters can inject into the hypothalamus include cues to the body temperature, blood and tissue oxygen levels, tissue water supplies, and glucose supplies.

Perhaps the easiest idea to manipulate is temperature. One way of persuading the brain that the body is being fed is to turn up body heat. Body heat can be increased by eating or drinking something hot or by putting on extra clothes and moving into a warm room.

Another way to trick the unfed hypothalamus is to persuade it that there is more oxygen in the tissues than is actually there. If a woman feels hungry, she should do some exercises.

The second line of defense against hunger is the gut. One way to trick the gut into feeling fed is to eat large amounts of low-calorie foods. This may not quench the fires of hunger, but it can make the dieter feel so full that she does not want food. Salads and vegetables are good for this purpose. So are soups and cereals. And the hotter the food the better.

The third line of defense against the gnawing desire for food is the endocrine system which pervades the whole body, reinforces the brain and the gut, and responds to certain general practices of controlling hunger.

The time it takes various food components to pass through the gut can be used to advantage by the dieter. The ideal meal plan for anyone with an ungovernable appetite is to start the meal with something sweet and follow it with a salad, then eat the rest of the meal.

Dieters who have trouble keeping their appetites in check at parties and gala dinners should prediet rather than postdiet. If a woman must overeat, she should do it on an empty stomach.

The frequent advice to drink plenty of water while one is on a diet is appropriate. Not only does the water make the stomach feel full, but whatever works to preserve fat store in the body seems closely related to whatever it is that conserves water.

Special attention should also be given to carbohydrate intake. Fat burns best and fastest in the presence of carbohydrates, and the dieter's own lean tissue is at risk when there is no starch or sugar coming into the system to provide fuel for burning fat. At least 50 percent of a well-balanced fat-reducing diet should be in the form of carbohydrates.

Mental and physical appetite control can be reinforced by social contacts that prove effective for many people. Group therapy often helps the dieter. Many people join Weight Watchers and similar organizations because they believe that support of others will strengthen their resolve. Some of the groups work on the same principle as Alcoholics Anonymous. When a dieter gets an urge to head for the refrigerator, he heads for the telephone instead and calls a fellow fatty.

DIET AND NUTRITION: HOW TO CHOOSE A DIET

BREAKFAST, 215 calories: 1 cup strawberries; 1 egg (large) cooked to own preference; 1 slice low-calorie bread or toast; 1 teaspoon low-calorie margarine or 1 tablespoon low-calorie jelly; no-calorie beverage.

LUNCH, 370 calories: ¾ cup cottage cheese; ½ cup green beans (boiled or raw); 4 fish sticks; 1 sliced tomato; ½ cup fresh pineapple slices; no-calorie beverage.

DINNER, 430 calories: ½ cup skim or low-fat milk; 4 oz. broiled lean beef steak; baked potato without skin; 1 tablespoon sour cream; ¼ cup blueberries.

TOTAL CALORIES: 1,015

CHAPTER 21
LOW-CALORIE MENUS AND RECIPES

Starvation crash diets are futile. The overfat woman who loses weight for a few weeks on a fad diet is unnecessarily torturing herself. When she returns to her old pattern of eating, her fat will come back with it.

It cannot be emphasized too often that calories and balance are the keys to a fat-reducing diet. A fat-reducing diet centered around calories and balance is the only suitable one for the treatment of obesity. A low-calorie balanced diet is the only one that is safe for a lifetime.

If a woman wants a slender body she must continue to eat the same food that reduced her. Such a commitment seems like a cruel life sentence, but there is compensation. She will look better and feel better. The same habit-forming mechanism that impelled her to overeat will eventually accustom her to the habits that keep her slender.

While all food groups are essential to the reducing diet, the groups vary in their fat-producing potential. There is even considerable variation within each group.

Those who are reducing should limit their fat intake. Some fat, both animal and vegetable, is necessary to health. The minimum amount of fats is required in a reducing diet. Very lean beef, pork, lamb, and other animal flesh is streaked with tiny, invisible filaments of fat. Those undetected filaments supply ample animal fat without butter, cream, or cheese. Chicken, turkey, other fowls, and all kinds of fish have very little fat, and they furnish the protein necessary to the body. For the reducing diet, therefore, fish and fowl are preferred to meat.

A potato has more calories than a turnip of the same size. Yet both should be eaten. A pound of chocolate candy has 2,395 calories. A pound of cabbage has 56. The secret of reducing is in eating very little of those foods high in calories and more of those low in calories.

The following pages offer menus for 30 days. Each menu totals approximately 1,000 calories. The small numbers at the top of some foods indicate that the recipes corresponding to those numbers will be found at the end of the chapter.

At the beginning of the reducing program, most of

the food portions should be weighed or measured.

The menus have been scientifically tested for calorie and nutrition content.

1

BREAKFAST, 210 calories: 1 orange or ½ cup orange juice; 1 egg (large) cooked to own preference (soft boiled, poached, or fried in no-calorie vegetable cooking spray); 1 slice low-calorie bread or toast; 1 teaspoon low-calorie margarine or 1 tablespoon low-calorie jelly; no-calorie beverage (coffee, tea, water, soda).
LUNCH, 400 calories: Summer Salad[1]; 1 slice low-calorie bread; 4 oz. turkey; ½ cup skim or low-fat milk.
DINNER, 400 calories: ¼ cup cottage cheese; ½ cup asparagus; ¼ cup cooked carrots; 1 slice whole wheat bread; ½ cantaloupe or honeydew melon; 4 oz. leg of lamb, lean; no-calorie beverage.
TOTAL CALORIES: 1,010

2

BREAKFAST, 270 calories: Grilled Swiss cheese sandwich (1 oz. Swiss cheese; 1 tablespoon low-calorie margarine spread on 1 side of 2 slices low-calorie bread; grill using no-calorie vegetable spray); 1 cup tomato or V-8 juice; no-calorie beverage.
LUNCH, 360 calories: 4 oz. lean ground hamburger; 1 slice low-calorie bread; 1 peach or plum; ½ cup boiled broccoli with 1 tablespoon lemon juice; no-calorie beverage.
DINNER, 370 calories: ½ cup skim or low-fat milk; 1 slice low-calorie bread; 10 raw or steamed oysters (medium size), cocktail sauce; 2 tablespoons baked apple; no-calorie beverage.
TOTAL CALORIES: 1,000

3

BREAKFAST, 210 calories: 1 oz. cold cereal or ⅓ cup (uncooked) oatmeal; ½ cup skim milk or low-fat milk; ½ grapefruit or ½ cup grapefruit juice; no-calorie beverage.
LUNCH, 395 calories: 4 oz. roast beef on 2 slices low-calorie bread with 1 teaspoon mustard; ½ cup asparagus; ½ cup strawberries; 1 oz. farmer or pot cheese; no-calorie beverage.
DINNER, 375 calories: 4 oz. roast turkey, meat only; ½ cup broccoli with 1 tablespoon lemon juice; 1 slice rye bread; ½ honeydew or cantaloupe melon; no-calorie beverage.
TOTAL CALORIES: 980

4

BREAKFAST, 205 calories: ½ cup diced pineapple; 1 slice honey ham loaf; 1 slice low-calorie bread or toast; 1 teaspoon low-calorie margarine or 1 tablespoon low-calorie jelly; ¼ cup cottage cheese; no-calorie beverage.
LUNCH, 385 calories: 3½ oz. tuna fish (oil packed drained); ½ cauliflower boiled or raw; 1 slice low-calorie bread; 1 banana; ½ cup skim or low-fat milk.
DINNER, 430 calories: 4 oz. roast beef, lean; 1 baked potato without skin; 1 tablespoon sour cream; 1 slice low-calorie bread; ½ cup strawberries; no-calorie beverage.
TOTAL CALORIES: 1,020

5

BREAKFAST, 255 calories: French Toast[2]; 1 teaspoon low-calorie margarine or 1 tablespoon low-calorie jelly; ½ cup apple juice; no-calorie beverage.

LUNCH, 315 calories: Spinach Salad[3]; 2 tablespoons Italian low-calorie salad dressing; 1 slice pumpernickel bread; 1 teaspoon low-calorie margarine; 2 slices bacon, cooked crisp; 5 prunes (dried); no-calorie beverage.

DINNER, 425 calories: 4 oz. veal loin chop or Veal Parmesan[4]; ⅓ cup tomato sauce; ½ oz. Mozzarella cheese; ½ cup cooked cabbage; ¼ cup fresh sliced pineapple; ½ cup skim or low-fat milk.
TOTAL CALORIES: 995

6

BREAKFAST, 250 calories: Dominique egg[5]; 1 orange or ½ cup orange juice; 1 small sliced tomato; no-calorie beverage.

LUNCH, 370 calories: Honeydew-Turkey Salad[6]; ½ cup cauliflower with paprika; 1 slice whole wheat bread; ½ cup skim or low-fat milk; no-calorie beverage.

DINNER, 380 calories: ½ cucumber, sliced; ¼ cup cottage cheese; 4 oz. flounder filet, with 1 tablespoon lemon juice; 1 slice rye bread; 1 ear of corn (medium size); 1 teaspoon low-calorie margarine; 1 apple; no-calorie beverage.
TOTAL CALORIES: 1,000

7

BREAKFAST, 235 calories: 1 cup tomato or V-8 juice; ½ cup flavored yogurt; 1 slice of low-calorie bread or toast; 1 teaspoon low-calorie margarine or 1 tablespoon low-calorie jelly; no-calorie beverage.

LUNCH, 355 calories: Beef Patty Parmesan[7]; Mushroom-Parsley Salad[8]; no-calorie beverage.

DINNER, 405 calories: ½ cup skim or low-fat milk; 4 oz. roast chicken, meat only; 1 cup spinach cooked with 2 tablespoons vinegar; 1 slice whole wheat bread; ¼ cup unsweetened apple sauce; no-calorie beverage.
TOTAL CALORIES: 995

8

BREAKFAST, 265 calories: 1 oz. cold cereal or ⅓ cup cooked oatmeal; ½ cup skim or low-fat milk; 1 banana; no-calorie beverage.

LUNCH, 370 calories: Cucumber-Tuna Salad[9]; 2 carrots in sticks; 1 slice pumpernickel bread; 1 cup strawberries; ½ cup skim or low-fat milk; no-calorie beverage.

DINNER, 365 calories: ½ can beef consomme; 2 oz. broiled beef liver; ½ cup cooked onions; 1 slice low-calorie bread; ½ cup mashed acorn squash; ½ cup grapes; no-calorie beverage.
TOTAL CALORIES: 1,000

DIET AND NUTRITION: LOW-CALORIE MENUS AND RECIPES

9

BREAKFAST, 215 calories: 1 cup strawberries; 1 egg (large) cooked to own preference; 1 slice low-calorie bread or toast; 1 teaspoon low-calorie margarine or 1 tablespoon low-calorie jelly; no-calorie beverage.

LUNCH, 370 calories: ¾ cup cottage cheese; ½ cup green beans (boiled or raw); 4 fish sticks; 1 sliced tomato; ½ cup fresh pineapple slices; no-calorie beverage.

DINNER, 430 calories: ½ cup skim or low-fat milk; 4 oz. broiled lean beef steak; baked potato without skin; 1 tablespoon sour cream; ¼ cup blueberries.

TOTAL CALORIES: 1,015

10

BREAKFAST, 255 calories: ½ cantaloupe or honeydew melon; ¼ cup cottage cheese; 2 slices bacon cooked crisp; 1 slice low-calorie bread or toast; 1 teaspoon low-calorie margarine or 1 tablespoon low-calorie jelly; no-calorie beverage.

LUNCH, 375 calories: Pineapple-Chicken Salad[10]; 2 lettuce leaves; 1 slice whole wheat bread; ½ cup skim or low-fat milk.

DINNER, 360 calories: 4 oz. steamed scallops; 1 slice pumpernickel bread; 1 tomato, broiled slices; ½ cup frozen French cut green beans; 1 sectioned orange with ¼ cup black raspberries; no-calorie beverage.

TOTAL CALORIES: 990

11

BREAKFAST, 210 calories: 1 apple; 1 oz. American processed cheese melted on 1 slice low-calorie bread (broiled); no-calorie beverage.

LUNCH, 365 calories: 4 oz. canned salmon; 1 slice low-calorie toast; 1 pear; ½ cup winter squash, mashed; no-calorie beverage.

DINNER, 415 calories: ½ cup skim or low-fat milk; ½ green pepper, sliced; ½ cup beets; ¾ cup broiled mushrooms; 1 slice whole wheat bread; 3 oz. fried beef liver; ½ cup cherries; no-calorie beverage.

TOTAL CALORIES: 990

12

BREAKFAST, 250 calories: Scrambled Egg Special[11]; 1 slice low-calorie bread or toast; 1 teaspoon low-calorie margarine or 1 tablespoon low-calorie jelly; ¼ cup fresh diced pineapple; no-calorie beverage.

LUNCH, 385 calories: 5 oz. loin lamb chop, broiled; ½ cup unsweetened apple sauce; 1 cup cauliflower (boiled or raw) with ¼ cup American cheese, melted; 1 slice pumpernickel bread; ½ green pepper; 5 radishes; ½ cup skim or low-fat milk.

DINNER, 365 calories: ¼ cup cottage cheese; ¾ cup hot V-8 juice; 3½ oz. broiled trout; 1 slice low-calorie bread; ½ cup cooked cabbage; no-calorie beverage.

TOTAL CALORIES: 1,000

13

BREAKFAST, 280 calories: Potato Pancakes[12]; 1 tablespoon sour cream; ½ cup tomato or V-8 juice; no-calorie beverage.

LUNCH, 360 calories: Oyster-Spinach Soup[13]; 5 saltine crackers; 1 tomato sliced, 2 oz. cottage cheese; no-calorie beverage.

DINNER, 360 calories: ½ cup skim or low-fat milk; Fried Chicken Special[14]; ½ cup asparagus; 1 tangerine, sectioned; no-calorie beverage.

TOTAL CALORIES: 1,000

14

BREAKFAST, 255 calories: 1 orange in sections; ½ cup blueberries; 1 oz. cold cereal or ⅓ cup (uncooked) oatmeal; ½ cup skim or low-fat milk; no-calorie beverage.

LUNCH, 255 calories: Shrimp cocktail (12 medium/large shrimp; 3 tablespoons cocktail sauce); Broccoli-Tomato Salad[15]; ½ cup green grapes; no-calorie beverage.

DINNER, 410 calories: ¼ cup cottage cheese with 1 peach, sliced; 4 oz. broiled chopped lean sirloin; 1 slice whole wheat bread; ½ tomato, sliced; no-calorie beverage.

TOTAL CALORIES: 920

15

BREAKFAST, 275 calories: Bacon Omelet[16]; 1 peach or plum; 1 slice low-calorie bread or toast; 1 teaspoon low-calorie margarine or 1 tablespoon low-calorie jelly; no-calorie beverage.

LUNCH, 390 calories: Tuna Salad[17]; 1 slice low-calorie bread; 1 teaspoon low-calorie margarine; ½ cup cooked sliced beets; 1 orange, sectioned; no-calorie beverage.

DINNER, 340 calories: ½ cup skimmed or low-fat milk; 1 slice honey ham loaf; Eggplant Parmesan[18]; 1 slice low-calorie bread; ½ cup cherries; no-calorie beverage.

TOTAL CALORIES: 1,005

16

BREAKFAST, 265 calories: ½ cup red raspberries (fresh or unsweetened) with 1 peach, sliced; ¼ cup cottage cheese; 2 slices low-calorie bread or toast; 2 tablespoons low-calorie jelly or 2 teaspoons low-calorie margarine; no-calorie beverage.

LUNCH, 370 calories; Grilled Swiss cheese sandwich (1 oz. Swiss cheese, 1 teaspoon low-calorie margarine; 2 slices low-calorie bread); Broccoli Soup[19]; 2 carrot and 2 celery sticks; no-calorie beverage.

DINNER, 370 calories: 4 oz. fish (red snapper); 1 tablespoon lemon juice; Mashed Potatoes[20]; ½ cup broiled mushrooms; ½ green pepper, sliced; 5 radishes; 1 banana; no-calorie beverage.

TOTAL CALORIES: 1,005

17

BREAKFAST, 285 calories: 1 oz. cold cereal or ⅓ cup (uncooked) oatmeal; 3 tablespoons raisins; ½ cup skim or low-fat milk; ½ cup fresh diced pineapple; no-calorie beverage.

LUNCH, 365 calories: 4 oz. fresh crabmeat; 1 tablespoon cocktail sauce; 1 cup blueberries; ½ cup frozen French cut beans (uncooked); 1 slice whole wheat bread; 2 oz. pot or farmer cheese; no-calorie beverage.

DINNER, 350 calories: 1 cup beef boullion with ¼ cup mushroom slices; ½ cup white rice; 4 oz. leg of lamb, lean; ½ cup cooked carrots, 1 sliced peach, no-calorie beverage.

TOTAL CALORIES: 1,000

18

BREAKFAST, 260 calories: Western Egg[21]; 1 slice low-calorie bread or toast; 1 teaspoon low-calorie margarine; ½ grapefruit, broiled; ½ tomato, sliced; no-calorie beverage.

LUNCH, 380 calories: 4 oz. broiled veal chop, fat removed; ½ cup asparagus; 1 slice low-calorie bread; ½ cup green grapes; no-calorie beverage.

DINNER, 360 calories: ½ can chunky clam chowder soup; 1 slice rye bread; 1 oz. pot cheese; 1 cup green beans; ½ cantaloupe; ½ cup skim or low-fat milk.

TOTAL CALORIES: 1,000

19

BREAKFAST, 265 calories: Grilled Swiss cheese sandwich (1 oz. Swiss cheese, 2 slices low-calorie bread, 1 teaspoon low-calorie margarine); no-calorie beverage.

LUNCH, 395 calories: Summer Salad (refer to recipe #1); 1 slice low-calorie bread; 4 oz. roast turkey (fat removed); ½ cup skim or low-fat milk.

DINNER, 350 calories: Raw vegetable salad (1 carrot in strips; 2 ripe olives; ½ cup cauliflower; 4 oz. chicken livers, simmered; with ½ cup mushrooms and ½ cup onions); ½ grapefruit; no-calorie beverage.

TOTAL CALORIES: 1,010

20

BREAKFAST, 265 calories: ½ grapefruit or ⅓ cup grapefruit juice; ¼ cup cottage cheese; 2 slices bacon cooked crisp; 1 slice low-calorie bread or toast; 1 teaspoon low-calorie margarine or 1 tablespoon low-calorie jelly; no-calorie beverage.

LUNCH, 395 calories: Shrimp Salad[22]; ½ can tomato soup (made with water), sprinkle ½ oz. Swiss cheese in soup; 1 slice low-calorie bread, toasted; ½ cup cherries; no-calorie beverage.

DINNER, 340 calories: 4 oz. roasted turkey; 1 slice rye bread; ½ cup broccoli with 1 tablespoon lemon juice; ½ honeydew or cantaloupe; no-calorie beverage.

TOTAL CALORIES: 1,000

21

BREAKFAST, 275 calories: 1 peach, sliced; 1 poached egg; Hash Brown Potatoes[23]; 1 slice low-calorie bread or toast; 1 teaspoon low-calorie margarine or 1 tablespoon low-calorie margarine or 1 tablespoon low-calorie jelly; no-calorie beverage.

LUNCH, 370 calories: ½ cup cottage cheese; ½ cup green beans; 1 slice low-calorie bread; 2 oz. liverwurst; 1 tomato, sliced; ½ cup fresh pineapple slices; no-calorie beverage.

DINNER, 355 calories: 8 oz. broiled clams with 2 tablespoons soy sauce; ½ cup white rice, ready to serve; ½ cup skim or low-fat milk; ½ cup cooked collard or other type greens.

TOTAL CALORIES: 1,000

22

BREAKFAST, 235 calories: ½ cup flavored yogurt; 1 slice low-calorie bread or toast; 1 teaspoon low-calorie margarine or 1 tablespoon low-calorie jelly; 1 cup tomato or V-8 juice; no-calorie beverage.

LUNCH, 400 calories: 3 oz. chicken; 1 tomato, sliced; 1 egg bagel; ½ cantaloupe or honeydew melon; ½ cup skim or low-fat milk.

DINNER, 365 calories: 3 oz. pork roast; ½ cup unsweetened applesauce; 1 cup yellow crook neck squash, sliced and cooked; ½ cup brussels sprouts; 1 tangerine, sectioned; no-calorie beverage.

TOTAL CALORIES: 1,000

23

BREAKFAST, 260 calories: 1 orange or ½ cup orange juice; 2 slices French Toast (see recipe #2); 1 teaspoon low-calorie jelly or cinnamon if desired; no-calorie beverage.

LUNCH, 370 calories: 3 oz. pork roast, lean only; Spinach Salad (refer to recipe #3); 2 tablespoons Italian salad dressing; 1 slice whole wheat bread; 1 teaspoon low-calorie margarine; ½ cup cherries; no-calorie beverage.

DINNER, 375 calories: ½ cup skim or low-fat milk; 2 oz. farmer or pot cheese; 1 slice rye bread; 4 oz. flounder filet, with 1 tablespoon lemon juice; 1 baked apple; ½ cup cooked peas; no-calorie beverage.

TOTAL CALORIES: 1,005

24

BREAKFAST, 275 calories: ½ cantaloupe or honeydew melon; 2 slices bacon, cooked crisp; 1 large egg, cooked to own preference; 1 slice low-calorie bread or toast; 1 teaspoon low-calorie margarine or 1 tablespoon low-calorie jelly; no-calorie beverage.

LUNCH, 365 calories: 4 oz. canned pink salmon, flaked over; 1 slice low-calorie toast; ½ cup winter squash, mashed; 1 banana; no-calorie beverage.

DINNER, 365 calories: ½ cup cottage cheese with 1 peach; ½ cup skim or low-fat milk; 1 slice whole wheat bread; 2 slices honey ham loaf; 1 carrot in strips; ¾ cup cooked cabbage; no-calorie beverage.

TOTAL CALORIES: 1,005

25

BREAKFAST, 260 calories: 1 banana; 1 oz. American processed cheese melted on 1 slice of low-calorie toast (broiled); ½ tomato, sliced; no-calorie beverage.

LUNCH, 370 calories: Honeydew-Turkey Salad (refer to recipe #6); 1 slice whole wheat bread; ½ cup asparagus; ½ cup skim or low-fat milk.

DINNER, 370 calories: 4 oz. broiled lean steak; 1 slice low-calorie bread toasted with 1 teaspoon low-calorie margarine; 1 cup lettuce, with 1 green pepper diced; ½ onion, diced; 4 radishes, sliced; 2 tablespoons Italian low-calorie dressing.

TOTAL CALORIES: 1,000

26

BREAKFAST, 245 calories: 1 Dominique Egg (refer to recipe #5) with 1 slice low-calorie bread and 1 teaspoon low-calorie margarine; 1 banana; no-calorie beverage.

LUNCH, 380 calories: 4 oz. roast beef on 2 slices low-calorie bread with 1 teaspoon mustard; ½ cup cooked carrots; ½ cup strawberries; no-calorie beverage.

DINNER, 370 calories: Eggplant Parmesan (refer to recipe #18); ½ cup skim or low-fat milk; 1 slice whole wheat bread; ½ cup cooked peas; ½ cup fresh diced pineapple.

TOTAL CALORIES: 995

27

BREAKFAST, 280 calories: Potato Pancakes (refer to recipe #12); top with ½ cup unsweetened applesauce, or 1 tablespoon sour cream; ½ cup tomato juice; no-calorie beverage.

LUNCH, 375 calories: Oyster-Spinach Soup (refer to recipe #13); Swiss cheese broiled (open face 1 oz.) on 1 slice low-calorie bread; ½ grapefruit; no-calorie beverage.

DINNER, 345 calories: ½ cup skim or low-fat milk; 3 oz. fried liver; ½ cup fried onions; 1 slice low-calorie bread; ½ cup asparagus.

TOTAL CALORIES: 1,000

28

BREAKFAST, 235 calories: 1 oz. cold cereal or ⅓ cup (uncooked) oatmeal; ½ cup red raspberries (fresh or unsweetened) with one sliced peach; ½ cup skim or low-fat milk; no-calorie beverage.

LUNCH, 395 calories: 5 oz. lamb chop broiled; ½ cup unsweetened applesauce; 1 baked potato without peel; 1 slice whole wheat bread; ½ cup beets; no-calorie beverage.

DINNER, 360 calories: 1 cup sauerkraut, drained; Bar-b-que Chicken[24]; 1 slice low-calorie bread; 1 oz. farmer or pot cheese; no-calorie beverage.

TOTAL CALORIES: 990

29

BREAKFAST, 265 calories: ½ cantaloupe or honeydew melon; 1 oz. cheddar cheese grilled with 2 slices low-calorie bread using 1 teaspoon low-calorie margarine; no-calorie beverage.

LUNCH, 370 calories: ½ cup mushrooms, sauted in 1 tablespoon low-calorie margarine; ½ cup raspberries mixed with 1 sectioned tangerine; no-calorie beverage.

DINNER, 365 calories: 4 oz. fresh crabmeat, with 1 tablespoon cocktail sauce; ½ cup frozen French cut beans; 1 cup blueberries; 1 slice whole wheat bread; ½ cup skim or low-fat milk.

TOTAL CALORIES: 1,000

30

BREAKFAST, 265 calories: Ham and Cheese Omelet[25]; 1 slice low-calorie bread or toast; 1 teaspoon margarine or 1 tablespoon low-calorie jelly; no-calorie beverage.

LUNCH, 375 calories: Shrimp cocktail (12 medium/large shrimp with 3 tablespoons cocktail sauce); Mushroom-Parsley Salad (refer to recipe #8); 1 slice pumpernickel bread; ½ cup skim or low-fat milk; ½ cup green grapes; no-calorie beverage.

DINNER, 335 calories: 4 oz. lean hamburger; 1 slice low-calorie bread; 2 leaves lettuce; ½ tomato; ¼ cup fresh diced pineapple; no-calorie beverage.

TOTAL CALORIES: 975

Low-Calorie Recipes

SUMMER SALAD[1]:

1 cup lettuce, shredded; 1 tomato, sliced; ¾ cup yellow crooked-necked squash, sliced; ¼ cup green onion, sliced; dressing -- 1 tablespoon salad seasonings, Italian spice seasoning, and salt and pepper, plus 2 tablespoons vinegar. Mix all vegetables together. Top with dressing.

FRENCH TOAST[2]:

Dip two slices of low-calorie bread in mixture of 1 beaten egg, pinch of cinnamon, ⅛ teaspoon vanilla extract, and artificial sweetener. Using no-calorie cooking spray, brown bread on both sides. Top with low-calorie margarine, low-calorie jelly, or more cinnamon.

SPINACH SALAD[3]:

1 cup torn spinach; ½ cup sliced mushrooms; ¼ cup sliced purple onions; 2 tablespoons toasted sesame seeds. Mix vegetables together. Sprinkle sesame seeds over top.

VEAL PARMESAN[4]:

4 oz. lean veal; ½ oz. Mozzarella cheese, sliced; 1/3 cup tomato sauce. Heat tomato sauce in saucepan using preferred seasoning. Fry veal in no-calorie cooking spray. When done, turn heat off, add cheese to veal, and cover until melted. Pour tomato sauce over top and serve.

DOMINIQUE EGG[5]:

Spread 1 slice low-calorie bread with 1 teaspoon low-calorie margarine. Cut a two-inch hole in middle of bread. In skillet, using no-calorie vegetable spray, brown both pieces of bread. Then crack egg into hole of bread and cook until ready. Top egg with circle of toast.

HONEYDEW-TURKEY SALAD[6]:

½ honeydew melon, cubed; ½ cup turkey, cubed; ½ cup celery, sliced; 1 tablespoon onion, diced; 2 tablespoons low-calorie French dressing. Mix ingredients and top with French dressing.

BEEF PATTY PARMESAN[7]:

4 oz. lean hamburger; ½ oz. Mozzarella cheese, sliced; 1/3 cup tomato sauce. Heat tomato sauce in pan using preferred seasoning. Fry hamburger in no-calorie cooking spray. When done, turn heat off, add cheese to burger, and cover until melted. Pour tomato sauce over top and serve.

MUSHROOM-PARSLEY SALAD[8]:

½ cup mushrooms, sliced; ⅛ cup parsley; ⅛ cup radishes, finely sliced; 1½ cups mixed greens (endive or bibb lettuce); pinch of basil, salt and pepper; 2 tablespoons low-calorie Italian dressing or wine vinegar. Combine ingredients, add seasoning, and top with dressing.

CUCUMBER-TUNA SALAD[9]:

1 small cucumber; 1/3 can or 2 oz. tuna fish; ¼ cup shredded processed American cheese; ⅛ cup chopped celery; 1 large hard-boiled egg, chopped; 1 tablespoon sweet pickle relish; 1 teaspoon onion, minced; ½ teaspoon lemon juice; paprika; salt and pepper. Cut cucumber in half length-wise and scrape out seeds. Cut a small slice from bottom of cucumber so it won't rock. Combine all ingredients and place in cucumber shells. Chill. Sprinkle with paprika and salt and pepper and serve. Makes 2 servings, 135 calories each.

PINEAPPLE-CHICKEN SALAD[10]:

½ cup chicken, cubed; ⅛ cup fresh pineapple, diced; ½ red-skinned apple, diced; ¼ cup celery, diced; 2 tablespoons raisins; salt and pepper; 1 tablespoon sour cream. Combine all ingredients, toss, and chill. Serve on salad greens.

SCRAMBLED EGG SPECIAL [11]:

1 large egg, beaten; 1 tablespoon skim or low-fat milk; 1 tablespoon green onion, sliced; 1 slice honey ham loaf (cut into bite-size pieces). Stir all ingredients together and scramble using no-calorie cooking spray.

POTATO PANCAKES [12]:

1 egg, beaten; 2 tablespoons skim or low-fat milk; 1 cup shredded potato; 2 tablespoons onion, diced; 1½ tablespoons flour; ¼ teaspoon salt; ⅛ teaspoon pepper. Combine egg and milk; add shredded potato and onion mix. Then add flour, salt, and pepper and mix well. Using large skillet or electric griddle and no-calorie cooking spray, drop mixture by the spoonful (Makes 3 to 4). Cook slowly until well browned and crisp. Turn and brown other side. Top with either sour cream or unsweetened applesauce.

OYSTER-SPINACH SOUP [13]:

1 cup skim or low-fat milk; 1 can condensed cream of chicken soup; 1, 10 oz. package frozen creamed spinach; 1, 8 oz. can of oysters, undrained; ½ cup dry white wine; pepper; lemon slices. In a large sauce pan stir milk into soup. Remove spinach from plastic pouch and add to soup. Cook and stir over medium heat, breaking up spinach until it is thawed. Simmer uncovered 10 minutes stirring occasionally. Stir in oysters, wine, and pepper. To serve, garnish with lemon slices. Makes 4 servings.

FRIED CHICKEN SPECIAL [14]:

½ chicken breast; salt and pepper; ⅛ cup bread crumbs. Season chicken breast with salt and pepper. Brown using no calorie cooking spray. Sprinkle half of bread crumbs on one side. Turn 5 minutes later and sprinkle the rest on. Cook until done.

BROCCOLI-TOMATO SALAD [15]:

1 cup fresh broccoli flowerets; 2 tablespoons sour cream; dash of curry powder, dry mustard, seasoned salt, and pepper; 1 tomato, sliced. Cook broccoli in boiling salted water 3 to 4 minutes. Let cool. Combine sour cream and seasoning; pour over broccoli and stir to coat. Chill 2 or 3 hours. Add sliced tomato and serve on lettuce leaves.

BACON OMELET [16]:

1 egg, large; 2 slices bacon, cooked crisp and cut up; 1 tablespoon green onion, sliced; 1 tablespoon water; ½ teaspoon Worcestershire sauce; ¼ cup fresh mushrooms, sliced. Beat egg and pour into pre-heated skillet (use no-calorie cooking spray). Allow to cook until egg starts to become firm. Add rest of ingredients and cook for about a minute; turn over and continue cooking until done.

TUNA SALAD [17]:

3½ oz. tuna fish, oil drained; ¼ cup chopped celery; ¼ cup onion, chopped; 3 tablespoons cocktail sauce. Combine all ingredients and blend. Serve on lettuce leaves.

EGGPLANT PARMESAN [18]:

¾ cup eggplant, sliced; ½ cup tomato sauce; 1 oz. Mozzarella cheese, thinly sliced. Place half of eggplant on bottom of casserole dish. Cover with half of sauce and half of cheese and repeat. Cook at 400 degrees for 20 minutes.

BROCCOLI SOUP [19]:

1, 10 oz. package of frozen broccoli; 1 can condensed cream of mushroom soup; 1 can of low-fat milk; ¼ cup dry white wine; ¼ teaspoon dried tarragon; salt and pepper. In a saucepan, cook broccoli according to directions, and drain. Add soup, milk, wine, tarragon, and salt and pepper. Heat thoroughly. Serves four.

MASHED POTATOES[20]

1 potato, boiled and sliced; ⅛ cup skimmed or low-fat milk. Mix together and top with 1 tablespoon low-calorie margarine and salt and pepper.

WESTERN EGG[21]:

Using no-calorie cooking spray in a skillet, heat a slice of honey ham loaf on one side. Turn to other side and top with egg. Fry together to desired doneness. Place on toasted bread.

SHRIMP SALAD[22]:

1½ cups torn lettuce; 6 medium shrimp, cooked, deveined, and halved; 1 medium tomato, cut in wedges; 1 hard-boiled egg, sliced; 1 tablespoon green onion, chopped; ½ tablespoon snipped parsley; 1 tablespoon pitted ripe olives, sliced. Place lettuce in bowl. Arrange shrimp, tomatoes, egg slices, and olives over top. Serve with low-calorie dressing.

HASH BROWN POTATOES[23]:

1 cup shredded potatoes; 2 tablespoons onion, diced; salt and pepper. Mix ingredients together and put in skillet sprayed with no-calorie cooking oil. Press potatoes flat and cook until browned. Turn over and brown other side.

BAR-B-QUE CHICKEN[24]:

4 oz. roasted chicken, meat only; ¼ cup bar-b-que sauce. Place chicken in narrow pan. Cook for 20 minutes at 350 degrees. Brush sauce on top and cook until done.

HAM AND CHEESE OMELET[25]:

1 egg, large; 1 slice honey ham loaf, cut into pieces; 1 tablespoon green onion, sliced; 1 tablespoon water; ½ teaspoon Worcestershire sauce; 1 small tomato, diced; ¼ cup cottage cheese. Beat egg and pour into pre-heated skillet (use no-calorie cooking spray). Allow to cook until egg starts to become firm. Add rest of ingredients and cook for about a minute; turn over and continue cooking until done.

Reminders for Food Addicts

1. Remember, there are no quick and easy ways to reduce body fat. The fatter you are the more difficult and longer-lasting your task will be.

2. Remind yourself constantly that you are self-indulgent and undisciplined.

3. Do not shield yourself from the truth about your obesity. You are fat because you want to be.

4. Do not blame your glands for your extra tonnage. Only in very rare cases is fat caused by glands.

5. Forget your obese ancestors. You are responsible for your own figure.

6. Bear in mind that eating patterns are a habit that must be broken by sheer will power.

7. Remember that the reducing diet must be strictly and constantly followed not only until the fat is lost but for the rest of your life.

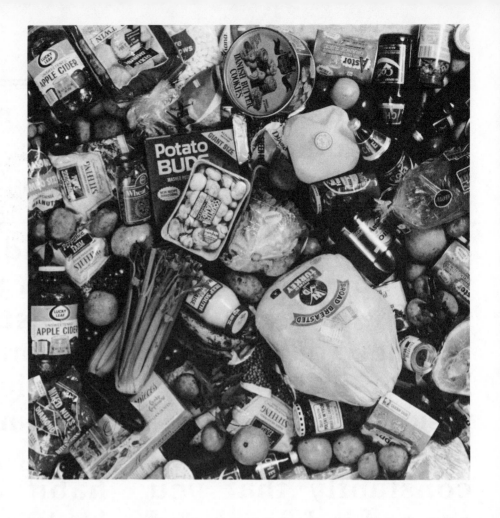

CHAPTER 22
EATING FOR FITNESS

There is a special group of fitness-minded women who, by the millions, are convinced that some miraculous elements are being removed from their food. Or that some government conspiracy is cold-bloodedly adding poisons to what they eat. And they are beginning to convince the people they come in contact with that there is indeed magic in their "health" foods, their "natural" eating, and their self-prescribed pills and supplements. Their rallying cry is that the supermarket shelves are stocked with what amounts to nutritional hemlock.

There is another group of women, primarily athletes, who are convinced that consuming certain food such as honey, wheat germ oil, or brewer's yeast, will improve performance. Other foods such as white bread, fried potatoes, and sugar, they say, should be avoided like the plague.

A small group of women, and a few men, in the home economics departments of the colleges and universities of the country have advanced degrees in nutrition. These usually quiet spoken, older women have for many years researched, applied, and taught nutrition. To them a well-balanced diet from a variety of foods purchased at the supermarket is all that is required for optimum nutrition.

What is a person to believe? What are the real facts about nutrition and its relationship to health and fitness?

The answers are not easy. The facts, in the scientific sense, have not all been discovered. Where the complex processes of the human body are concerned, it is impossible to understand everything about nutrition. Individual judgements have to be made. The final test, say some philosophers, is in the senses of the individual. Two people can be exposed to the same information and come away with opposite beliefs.

A person is most likely to believe what she has experienced. It would be fairly simple for women to have clear-cut beliefs about nutrition if the effects could be felt immediately. If, on a given day, a woman skipped her food source for vitamin C and felt lousy, and on another day she got vitamin C and felt great, she might not ask for scientific proof of the value of vitamin C.

Of course, nutritional effects are not that dramatic because they do not express themselves immediately as something felt or seen. The changes come gradually and may take months or even years. The source of individual beliefs then is intellectual, rather than physical. It is in the mind rather than in the bones and muscles.

Few people conduct their own experiments or do research to seek out facts about food and nutrition. Most of them learn from information others provide. Making sense out of words about food and nutrition is a matter of deciding **whom** to believe as well as **what** to believe.

SOME BASES
FOR JUDGING

On what do experts agree? Thousands of persons in the world give special study to nutrition:

researchers, biochemists, physicians, dieticians, and teachers. Their professional careers bring them into the mainstream of knowledge about food and nutrition. They do not agree on everything. But there is consensus on one general point: The best and simplest general nutrition advice today is that a person eat, in moderation, a wide variety of foods from each of the four basic groups.

When information suggests something much different from that base, a woman should weigh that information carefully. The proponent has departed from the basic agreement of professionals in the field.

A second basic agreement is that life is a balance of risks and benefits. Absolute safety is impossible. A woman must look at the benefits and risks, then decide where the balance is acceptable. Charcoaling meat may present a slight risk of cancer. Is that risk important enough to cause an individual to forgo the social benefits of outdoor cooking plus the charcoal flavor? Each individual must answer that question.

Much of what is known today about eating for fitness can be presented briefly and succinctly in a fallacy-fact discussion based on scientific evidence.

CALORIES

Fallacy: Fitness-minded women should not be concerned about calories.
Fact: Calories do count, every one of them. If a woman consumes more calories than her body expends, she will assuredly gain fat. If she consumes fewer calories than she needs, she will lose fat. The energy level of food eaten, minus the energy lost in the excreta, must equal the sum of the heat given off and the physical work done by the body. The unit measure of heat is the calorie, but few people know what a calorie really is.

A calorie is the amount of heat needed to raise the temperature of one liter of water one degree centigrade. A hundred calories would raise the temperature of one liter of water from the freezing to the boiling point.

WHEAT GERM OIL

Fallacy: Large doses of wheat germ and wheat germ oil will improve a woman's stamina.
Fact: Wheat germ is the most nutritious part of the wheat plant. It is often destroyed during the milling of the wheat flour. It is a rich source of B vitamins, protein, and vitamin E and can be eaten in a number of ways. When toasted, wheat germ becomes a tasty cereal with a nut-like flavor. When used as oil it can be eaten in salads. Some athletes drink the oil straight from the bottle. The problem with such foods is that unmilled whole grains and oils easily turn rancid and moldy if they are not refrigerated.

Some people claim that wheat germ can prevent aging, muscular dystrophy, and heart disease, as well as make a person more sexually potent. Many athletes believe that wheat germ oil increases their strength and endurance. None of these claims for wheat germ as a unique supplier of some essential therapeutic ingredients has been substantiated. Wheat germ and wheat germ oil are not essential foods. They are not unique or magic. Enriched flour, fruits, vegetables, meat, dairy products, and many other foods supply the same nutrients found in wheat germ.

HONEY AND QUICK ENERGY

Fallacy: Honey provides quick energy.
Fact: There are no quick-energy foods. Nor is there any magic in eating honey. Honey contains glucose and fructose, the same simple sugars that are produced by the digestion of table sugar. Honey contains a higher percentage of fructose, but it is not significantly superior to other common sweets. Unfortunately, some misinformed people have falsely promoted honey as a sweet that is better tolerated than other sugars.

Taken in large quantities, honey can produce several detrimental effects. Excessive amounts of honey, or other sweets, can draw fluid from other parts of the body into the gastrointestinal tract. This shift in fluids can dehydrate a woman in endurance-type activities where sweat loss can affect performance. A concentrated sugar solution may also distend the stomach, causing nausea, cramps and/or diarrhea. If a woman is determined to take honey or sugar, she should do so in small quantities with plenty of water. She should have no more than three tablespoons of sweets in any one-hour period. This will appease her physiological need. It will not improve her performance.

FRIED POTATOES

Fallacy: Fried poatoes are harmful to the digestive tract.
Fact: Greasy foods are digested slowly because fat retards the emptying time of the stomach, but this does no harm to a normal digestive tract. Most fats are digested at about the same rate whether they are in butter, margarine, salad dressing, shortening, or cooking oils used to fry foods. As for potatoes, they are one of the most nutritious vegetables. Fried potatoes are certainly not taboo for women.

HAMBURGERS

Fallacy: Hamburgers should be avoided during training.
Fact: A hamburger with all the trimmings is a fairly well-balanced meal. There is no good reason why fitness-minded people cannot eat hamburgers several times a week. People who eat regularly at fast-food chains, however, would be wise to make sure their other meals include enough fruits, vegetables, and dairy products. They should also keep in mind that fast-food hamburgers tend to be a bit too heavy in fat content.

BREAD

Fallacy: Bread is a fattening food which weight-conscious women should not consume.
Fact: Bread is one of the most nutritious foods that women can eat. It is low in calories, about 60 per slice, and contains ample amounts of niacin, riboflavin, thiamin, iron, protein, carbohydrates, and calcium. The real reason the majority of people relate bread to fattening food is not the bread itself, but what they put on it.

Fallacy: Individuals should avoid white bread. Only whole-grain breads should be eaten.
Fact: Basically, there are no significant differences between the nutritional quality of whole-grain bread and enriched white bread, especially when the cost of a loaf of each is considered. Enriched white bread, when thiamin, niacin, riboflavin, and iron have been added, and when milk solids are used in baking, provides practically the same vitamins and minerals as whole-wheat bread. It also gives twice as much riboflavin, and much more calcium because milk is lacking in whole-wheat bread. It is true that minute amounts in of some nutrients such as sodium, magnesium, and other trace elements are lost in milling white flour, but there are numerous other food sources of those lost nutrients.

Whole-grain breads are a fair source of fiber, which many authorities feel is helpful to bowel function. Women should eat whatever bread appeals to them.

BEE POLLEN

Fallacy: Bee pollen tablets offer a tremendous breakthrough in helping a woman obtain greater endurance.
Fact: The athletic world can thank the Finns for publicizing bee pollen. It all started in 1972 when Finland's Lasse Viren won the 5,000 and 10,000 meter runs in Munich and began buzzing the news about pollen tablets. When Viren repeated his successes in Montreal in 1976, health-food companies decided to increase the availability of bee pollen -- at a cost of $45 per pound.

The cost is a result not only of its supposed magical properties, but also the way it is harvested. As bees obtain nectar from flowers, pollen collects on their bodies. When they return to their hives, the pollen is scraped off by wire brushes that have been placed around the entrances. The very fine-grained powder is then collected and manufactured into tablets. According to the major U.S. distributor, bee pollen tablets contain all of the essential amino acids and many vitamins and minerals. None of these nutrients offer any magic, and all can be obtained easily and less expensively in conventional foods.

Recent research at Louisiana State University showed that bee pollen has no effect on the performance of runners and swimmers. When confronted with this evidence, the American distributor noted that the LSU study used bee pollen from France, not the full-potency pollen from England which, naturally, he sold. He also admitted that bee pollen is necessary when the diet is already well-balanced.

BREWER'S YEAST

Fallacy: Brewer's yeast is good for pep and energy.

Fact: Brewer's yeast is a bitter yellow powder related to a variety of yeast which is a by-product of beer brewing. It contains large amounts of B vitamins, amino acids, and minerals. Supplementing the diet with dried brewer's yeast might be useful if a woman is deficient in protein and B vitamins. But eating brewer's yeast is not the most effecient or the most appetizing way to obtain these nutrients. Besides, only vitamins obtainable by a prescription contain B vitamins in high enough doses to be therapeutically valuable.

YOGURT

Fallacy: Women with digestive problems should consume yogurt each day.

Fact: Yogurt is a fermented milk product and, like all dairy products, is an excellent source of protein and calcium. To say, however, that yogurt will help digestive problems is misleading. For those women who have an allergic reaction to the lactose in milk, yogurt may be helpful. The same thing can be said of buttermilk, which has almost equal nutrition value to that of yogurt and is considerably less expensive. In the 1950's and 1960's many health food faddists claimed that yogurt contained beneficial bacteria that assisted intestinal function. This has been proved false.

LECITHIN

Fallacy: Taking lecithin regularly is a preventative measure against heart disease.

Fact: Lecithin is the natural emulsifier found in egg yolk and soybeans and is sold in capsule and powder form at health food stores. It has long been publicized in health magazines as an antidote to high blood cholesterol and heart disease. Evidence shows that lecithin cannot dissolve the plaques in the blood vessels that contribute to heart attacks. Solving the problems associated with high blood cholesterol concentrations and heart attacks is much more complex than a simple feeding of lecithin to the patient.

RAW EGGS

Fallacy: Raw eggs can be added to a milk shake for additional nutrition.

Fact: Although the addition of raw eggs can improve the flavor and nutritional value of a milk shake, this should be avoided because of the possibility of illness from contaminated eggs. Residual salmonella organism, which causes food poisoning, can remain on the ouside of eggs even after washing. Invisible cracks in the shell may permit passage of the disease organism. Nutritionally, raw eggs are less desirable because they contain avidin which is neutralized in cooking. Avidin in an uncooked egg destroys the B vitamin, biotin. For milk shakes it is possible to use a slightly soft boiled egg to make a more nutritious drink.

PRE-COMPETITION MEALS

Fallacy: Pre-competition meals for women athletes should consist of special foods.

Fact: Although it may give a woman athlete a feeling of strength and security, what she eats on the day of competition has very little to do with the production of energy for that day. Women who compete in non-stop, marathon-type events are an exception to this rule. They can benefit from pre-event meals of carbohydrate-rich foods, as well as several days of carbohydrate loading. Nutritional scientists have found that it takes from two to fourteen days for the food a person eats to be utilized for energy. The following guidelines should be considered in planning pre-competition meals:

1. Energy intake should be adequate to ward off any feelings of hunger during competition.
2. The necessity for urinary or bowel excretion during competition can be serious or even

disabling. For this reason, large amounts of protein foods, bulky foods, or highly spiced foods should be avoided.

3. The meal should be eaten at least three hours prior to competition to allow for digestion.

4. Fluid intake before, during, and after prolonged competition should guarantee optimal hydration. This can be accomplished with water and various fruit juices.

5. The pre-competition meal should be food to which the woman is accustomed to eating. Food that gives her psychological assurance will strengthen her determination to win.

STEAK

Fallacy: Steak is the food of champions.

Fact: Thick, juicy steaks have been a training table staple for many years. This was especially prevalent during the 1950's and 1960's. Even today, many fitness-minded people believe that there is a corollary between red meat and strength and endurance.

Scientific research has repeatedly shown that steak, which contains protein and fat, is not as efficient in supplying energy for performance as food rich in carbohydrates. The ideal diet for most fitness-minded women should be 59 percent carbohydrates, 28 percent fats, and 13 percent proteins.

PROTEIN FOODS

Fallacy: Large amounts of protein foods and protein supplements are especially important during intense training.

Fact: The average woman in the United States consumes 104 grams of protein a day, more than twice her recommended requirement. Yet there are absolutely no health or performance benefits from consuming excessive protein foods. The following table was developed from the Recommended Dietary Allowances (RDA) of the Food and Nutrition Board of the National Research Council.

Fallacy: Protein foods are great for promoting power-packed energy.

Fact: The promotion of "power-packed" protein is a sales gimmick. Although proteins can be used as energy sources if necessary, carbohydrates and fats are preferable. They are used more easily by the body and also cost less than protein foods.

Fallacy: High-protein diets are a must for fat reduction.

Fact: Proteins and carbohydrates both have four calories per gram. Fats have nine calories per gram. Since high-protein foods (such as steaks) can contain a high percentage of fat, a high-protein reducing diet may actually have 70 percent or more of its calories coming from fat.

	Average Weight	For Protein Needed Multiply Weight by:	Average Protein Needed
Child, 1-3	28 pounds	0.80	22 grams
Child, 4-6	44 pounds	0.70	31 grams
Child, 7-10	66 pounds	0.55	36 grams
Male, 11-14	97 pounds	0.45	44 grams
Male, 15-18	134 pounds	0.40	54 grams
Male, over 19	162 pounds	0.36	58 grams
Female, 11-14	97 pounds	0.45	44 grams
Female, 15-18	119 pounds	0.40	48 grams
Female, over 19	135 pounds	0.36	49 grams

DIET AND NUTRITION: EATING FOR FITNESS

Part of the weight loss on a high-protein diet is caused by minor nausea and loss of appetite which lead to reduced caloric intake. As proteins are broken down, their waste products are flushed out of the body by the kidneys. The resultant water loss, perhaps five to eight pounds in the first week, may mislead the dieter into thinking she is losing fat. There is very little water in fat. The water actually comes from muscles, vital organs, and fluid ouside the cells. This is what takes place with the use of liquid protein supplements, amino acid supplements, and high-protein powders that are currently so popular. None of them cause long-term fat loss, and many are actually dangerous.

Fallacy: Large amounts of protein cannot hurt the body.
Fact: Scientists have recently found that too much dietary protein can be dangerous. The metabolism and excretion of nonstorable protein can impose serious stress and cause enlargement of the liver, kidneys, and other vital organs.

Government investigators believe that more than 50 deaths are linked to the combination of fasting plus low-quality protein supplements. A diet of this type was popularized by Dr. Robert Linn in his book, **The Last Chance Diet,** which was published in July 1976. Prior to this date, athletes, particularly bodybuilders and weightlifters, had been consuming liquid protein supplements for years. Fortunately, they were eating other foods. Scientists who have analyzed the dark syrupy liquids say they contain low-quality, partly digested protein derived from cattle hides and tendons. Artifical flavor is added to disguise the otherwise horrid taste.

There is no scientific evidence supporting the belief that fitness-minded people require massive amounts of protein-rich foods, protein supplements, or liquid amino acids.

ORGANICALLY GROWN FOOD

Fallacy: Fitness-minded women should try their best to eat organically grown fruits and vegetables.
Fact: Many women mistakenly believe that all organic foods are produced without pesticides and artificial fertilizers free of preservatives, hormones, and antibiotics. There are no legal standards concerning organically grown foods. There is not even a consistent definition of "organic" when applied to foods. "Organic" is not a synonym for "pure." The organic fertilizers of animal or human origin are the most likely to contain gastrointestinal parasites. Salmonella, which upsets more stomachs than probably anything else, is a frequent inhabitant of the gastrointestinal tract of animals and men. It represents a serious threat to the whole concept of organically grown foods, especially if the foods are not washed or cooked prior to consumption. The major danger in eating is still bacterial or parasitic contamination.

Fallacy: Richer soil makes food richer in vitamins.
Fact: The nutritive value of a food is determined primarily by the heredity in its seed. Thus, if minerals that are demanded by the plant's heredity are missing from the soil, the plant simply will not grow. If such minerals are scant in the soil, fewer plants will grow. The farmer whose soil lacks what plants need will soon be out of business.

Vitamins in foods are manufactured in the plants themselves by genetically controlled processes. The very fact that a fruit or vegetable exists is evidence that it has those nutrients essential for its growth.

There are trace minerals such as iodine that accumulate in the plant as it grows. These may or may not be part of its own food needs. Soils high or low in iodine tend to produce plants that are high or low in this mineral. Special techniques of cultivation such as organic farming do not solve this problem. It can be solved only by adding the necessary mineral element to the soil or the food. Organic foods have no value beyond the value of ordinary supermarket foods.

VITAMIN AND MINERAL PILLS

Fallacy: It is a good idea to take a multiple vitamin and mineral supplement every day.

Fact: A typical television commercial shows a slim, attractive woman explaining how she stays healthy. She says she watches her diet, gets plenty of exercise and "just to be sure" takes a daily vitamin-mineral supplement. The advertisement implies that a balanced diet cannot provide adequate enough nutrients. This is untrue. All necessary nutrients are easily obtained from a sensible diet of ordinary foods. The sole exception is that some women who have excessively heavy menstrual periods may need to take iron supplements.

Fallacy: Extra vitamins and minerals will make a woman feel less tired.

Fact: Vitamins are not medicines. The confusion here comes from the knowledge that serious vitamins or mineral deficiencies lead to symptoms and that restoring the missing nutrients to the diet relieves the symptoms. Once adequate vitamins and minerals are included in the diet of normal people, supplements rarely have a beneficial effect. The vast majority of illnesses that afflict Americans cannot be prevented or cured by extra vitamins and minerals. Neither can fatigue or that general tired feeling be assuaged by them.

VITAMIN C

Fallacy: Vitamin C tablets can ward off winter colds.

Fact: The value of vitamin C in preventing colds is still controversial. Most nutrition experts note, however, that massive doses can cause diarrhea, excessive urination, and kidney and bladder stones. They question its value in preventing colds. Until more conclusive evidence is available, women need not consume more than the normal daily vitamin C requirement. This requirement is easily obtainable from four servings of fruits and vegetables.

As research continues, there will be more knowledge about how much is too much of a vitamin, what the entire scope of usefulness of each vitamin is, and which medical conditions may respond well to vitamin therapy. In the meantime, exercise minded women should know that elaborate testimonials, miraculous claims, and vitamins supposedly derived from exotic sources result from mere guesswork, confusion, and often outright fraud.

NATURAL VERSUS SYNTHETIC VITAMINS

Fallacy: Vitamin pills from natural sources are preferable to synthetic ones.

Fact: Basically, there is no difference between natural and synthetic vitamins, except for the higher costs of the natural ones. Both have the same atoms in their molecules and are arranged in exactly the same way, which means their chemical activity is identical. A vitamin is a vitamin.

FRESH FRUITS AND VEGETABLES

Fallacy: Fresh fruits and vegetables are nutritionally superior to frozen or canned fruits and vegetables.

Fact: If "fresh" means locally grown, picked when ripe, and rushed to the market, this statement is not a fallacy. But if "fresh" means harvested in California and shipped by truck to the East Coast, canned or frozen produce is probably a better choice. Canned, frozen, and fresh, each in its own way and its own season has some advantages and disadvantages. The best way to ensure proper nutrition is to eat a wide variety of all kinds of fruits and vegetables whether they are canned, frozen or fresh.

CHEMICAL ADDITIVES

Fallacy: Chemical additives to food are detrimental to health.

Fact: All nutrients and all life are chemistry. An orange is a mixture of some 225 chemical compounds. When an individual eats an orange, the orange is broken down into chemicals. What happens now is a process of choosing. The body uses the chemicals it can and eliminates those it cannot.

The body does not choose between chemicals based upon whether they have chemical-sounding or natural-sounding names. Those prejudices exist in the mind, not the digestive system. The digestive system does care about two things: what the chemical is and how much of it is there.

Recently, the term "chemical" has come to stand for what is man-made. There has been the sad misunderstanding that what is natural is safe and what is man-made is potentially harmful. This has led to much needless worry and often too much exploitation of the consumer.

In reality, food additives are far safer than many natural components in foods. Carrots contain myristicin, a hallucinogen. Radishes contain goitrogens which promote goiter by interfering with our use of iodine. Potatoes have solanine which in great enough quantities can cause drowsiness, paralysis, or breathing problems. Shrimp have some 40 to 170 or more parts per million of arsenic. Similar chemicals can be found in all foods. There is potential danger in too much of any one food.

The foods found in the average home are not dangerous when consumed as a normal part of a balanced and varied diet. Eaten in moderation, they are all nutritious and safe.

SUGAR

Fallacy: Table sugar should be avoided like the plague.
Fact: Although refined sugar is a concentrated form of calories, it does not contain a single harmful substance. Nutritionists would prefer that women get most of their carbohydrates from fruits, vegetables, breads, and other foods that also supply vitamins, minerals, and bulk. Table sugar need not be avoided, but should be used in moderation.

FIBER

Fallacy: High-fiber diets can cure many aches and pains.
Fact: Dietary fiber, bran in particular, is being promoted as good for almost everything that ails people from constipation to heart disease. High-fiber cookbooks are on the increase. So are the high-fiber foods on supermarket shelves . Yet to the scientists who are investigating the effect of dietary fiber, the situation is far from clear. There are only two areas of general agreement.

A diet high in fiber plays a role in the prevention of constipation and diverticulitis. Diverticulitis is a disease caused by abnormal sacs or protrusions on the walls of the intestines. Dietary fiber by itself probably has no effect on cancer of the colon or coronary disease, or other disease of a less serious nature.

Before a woman buys a high-fiber supplement such as bran, she should examine her present diet. Food fiber comes in hundreds of different varieties, not in bran alone. Whole wheat bread contains fiber. So do broccoli, raw cabbage, apples, pineapples, carrots, and whole kernel corn.

Authorities differ in their recommendations for food fiber. Intake of crude fiber among Americans is about four grams per day. The individual intake in some non-industrialized countries is as much as 30 grams. Most people should have amounts somewhere between those figures.

A daily diet ample in fruits and vegetables as well as breads and cereals should provide a person with all she needs of useful fiber. Supplementary crude fiber is best obtained from certain breakfast cereals such as Kellogg's All Bran, Bran Buds, and Nabisco's 100% Bran.

SALT TABLETS

Fallacy: Women athletes should consume several salt tablets each day during hot weather.
Fact: Salt tablets usually do more harm than good. Women need more salt during hot weather, but salt tablets often irritate the stomach or pass through the system without being absorbed. Dr. Lawrence Lamb recommends that in addition to drinking plenty of water, athletes should drink at least a quart of low-fat milk or fortified skim milk a day, plus two eight-ounce glasses of orange juice. Milk has about the same salt content as the healthy human body, and orange juice contains potassium, which is also important in hot weather. A liberal use of the salt shaker during meals is usually sufficient for extra salt.

WATER

Fallacy: Drinking water during exercise will upset a woman's stomach.

Fact: Prohibiting water in the training room or on the practice field has no physiological basis. Withholding liquids during hot, humid weather makes a woman susceptible to heat cramps, heat exhaustion, or the more serious and sometimes fatal heat stroke. Dehydration causes fatigue, which in itself makes a woman more vulnerable to injury. All coaches, athletes, and exercise-minded people should realize the necessity of drinking fluids before, during and after vigorous activity. Furthermore, the fluids should be iced. The old idea that people warm from exercise should not drink ice water because it causes cramps is completely unfounded.

THE
LAST WORD

Good health, with its promise of vim and vigor, is a desirable state. The term "health" is often confused with "nutrition" and "fitness," however. To say that health and fitness are directly related to food is a misconception. Health and fitness are the result of many factors, just one of which is nutrition.

The body does not require any particular food. It uses some 50 nutrients in varying amounts. No nutrient is considered to be a health or fitness nutrient. But any nutrient is required for human nutrition is essential to life, health, and fitness, even though some are needed in very small amounts.

There are not fitness foods. Neither are there junk foods. Any food can be good if it is consumed in moderation with a variety of other foods. Any food can be bad if it is exclusively consumed.

The latest scientific research in fitness nutrition is still centered on a well-balanced diet. A well-balanced diet is all that is needed for optimum nutrition.

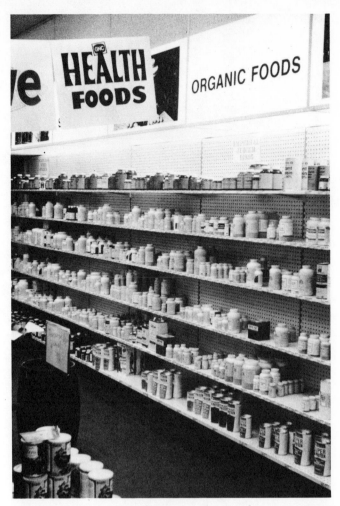

To say that health is directly related to food is a misconception. Health is a result of many factors, just one of which is food.

DIET AND NUTRITION: EATING FOR FITNESS

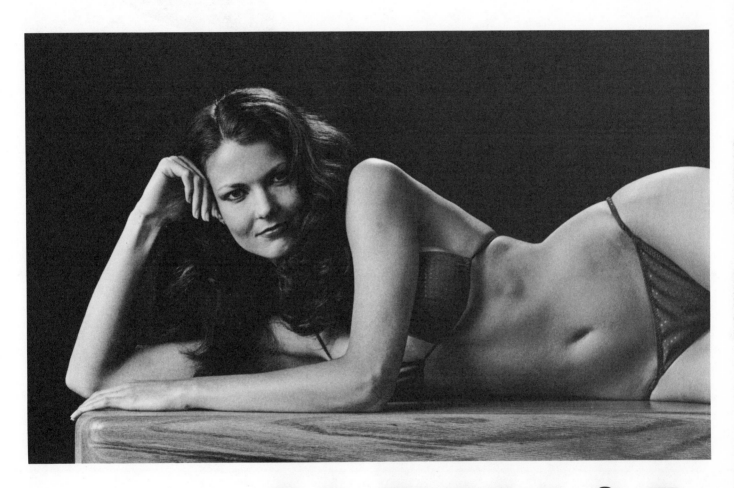

V. FINAL
TOUCHES

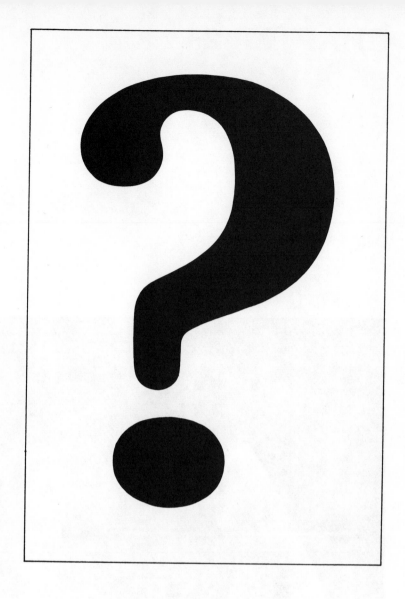

CHAPTER 23
QUESTIONS & ANSWERS

Q. What is resistance?

A. When performing body-shaping exercises, a woman produces force by contracting her muscles. To tax her contracting muscles she applies the weight of her body, air, water, cans, dumbbells, barbells, or whatever else she finds convenient against the force of her muscles. This counterforce or weight is known as resistance.

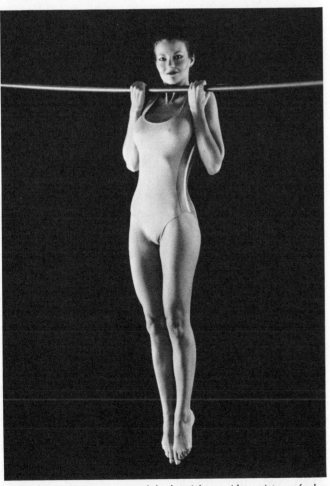

In the chinup exercise a woman's bodyweight provides resistance for her arm and torso muscles.

Q. In performing a specific body-shaping exercise, how does a woman know when her muscles have reached the point of fatigue?

A. All body-shaping exercise should be performed throughout a full range of motion -- smoothly and slowly without sudden, jerky movements. Assuming this rule is closely followed, movements are continued until proper execution becomes impossible. At this point fatigue is reached. Most women will experience a burning sensation several repetitions preceding fatigue in a given exercise. This sensation is normal and should be tolerated to obtain best results.

As a woman becomes stronger and shaplier, her exercises will become progressively strenuous.

If they do not become more strenuous, she is wasting much of her effort.

Q. How does a woman judge her progression?

A. A woman must keep accurate records of her exercises. She should record the exercise, repetitions, form, sequence, date, bodyweight, and any other factors she can measure.

Charting progress greatly assists a woman to assess her fatigue in the exercises and improvement in the program. If records indicate that 10 repetitions of an exercise are performed on a Monday, she can set her sights for 11 or 12 on the following Wednesday. Without encouraging records, she has no objectives to aim for.

FINAL TOUCHES

Q. When perfoming body-shaping exercises, how warm should the environment be?
A. When muscles contract they utilize energy. Part of this energy is released in the form of heat dissipated through the skin with the help of the vascular system. If the body comes becomes too hot, certain organs, especially the brain, can malfunction. To prevent this, a cool place to perform exercises is highly recommended. A temperature of between 65 and 75 degrees F is desirable.

Q. Is it beneficial to sweat when exercising?
A. When exercising, the body produces heat in proportion to the amount of muscular activity. The body's temperature could easily rise as much as ten degrees F or more, if this heat were not dissipated. Fortunately, the body is designed to keep itself from overheating. Warm blood is brought to the skin where it loses heat to the surrounding air. The sweat glands begin to secrete water, and the body is further cooled by evaporation of the perspiration. In cold weather, heat is given off easily. But in hot weather the body must sweat profusely in order to cool itself.

Sweating does not do anything but lower the body temperature. It does not help reduce body fat. The body may weigh less after a workout, but this is due to loss of water, and there is very little water in fat. As soon as thirst is satisfied, the body will regain the lost weight.

Sweating does not clean out the pores of the skin. There is no evidence that it is of any value in removing toxic materials from the body. Women should avoid rubber sweat suits, belts, wraps, and steam and sauna baths. They can contribute to heat stroke and high-blood pressure.

Sweating does not promote fitness. Fitness is developed by exercising the muscles of the body - not the sweat glands.

Q. Will body shaping help or hinder arthritis problems?
A. Arthritis is inflammation of the joints. It is found in a variety of manifestations. Body shaping will help most forms of arthritis, but some may respond adversely to any activity whatsoever. Any woman with such a condition should consult her physician.

Q. What exercises should be performed by a woman with low-back pain?
A. Low-back pain has numerous possible causes and symptoms. If it does not irritate a given condition, exercise should benefit anyone with back pain. But performed improperly, or for the wrong condition, exercise may adversely affect certain back ailments. To be absolutely sure, medical consultation is strongly recommended before beginning a body-shaping program if a woman already suffers from such a problem.

Q. What happens to a woman's bones when she becomes stronger?
A. When a muscle is strengthened, other body structures strengthen proportionally. This includes the muscle sheath, tendons, ligaments, and even bones.

Q. How does body shaping affect the brain?
A. While research definitely proves that body-shaping benefits the body, recent findings suggest that body shaping plays an important role in improving mental performance. Studies have shown that body shaping can increase the oxygen-transport capacity to all parts of the body, including the brain. Early research demonstrated that brain cells deprived of sufficient oxygen do not perform their work efficiently. The intellect and reasoning powers fail as a result. These studies demonstrate that a program of regular body shaping which increases oxygen transport to the brain can significantly improve mental performance. For optimum results, however, body shaping should be varied and challenging, and not just routine and repetitious.

Q. What is cardiovascular training?
A. Cardiovascular training is a program designed to improve the functional efficiency of the heart and the entire vascular system. This includes the heart, arteries, veins, capillaries, and even the chemical processes occurring at the cellular level in the working muscle.

Cardiorespiratory training is a program that trains all of the above mentioned and also includes the lungs. Cardiorespiratory and cardiovascular training are inseparable.

Q. Is a supplemental activity for cardiovascular training necessary in a body-shaping program?
A. Body-shaping exercises directly work the skeletal muscles and indirectly work the heart. This is basically true of all physical exercise.

The indirect involvement of the heart is dependent upon two factors:
1. The extent of muscular participation in each exercise
2. The quantity of rest allowed between each exercise

Maximum cardiovascular work will be evidenced if a woman exercises large muscular structures and rests little between and during activities. Average maximum heart rate is 220 minus her age. If she can sustain her heart rate at 75 percent of its maximum for 10 minutes or more three times per week she will experience cardiovascular improvement.

Q. Should a woman's conditioning program differ from that of a man?
A. There is no valid reason that a woman should exercise differently from a man. Hormones and genetic attributes will not permit the same results. A man will grow to look more as **he** should; a woman will grow to look more as **she** should. But the general programs should be the same.

Q. What makes a man's muscles grow?
A. In men, muscular growth occurs in two parts. One, there must be growth stimulation within the body at the basic cellular level. After puberty, this is best accomplished by high-intensity exercise. Two, the proper nutrients must be available for the stimulated cells. Large amounts of nutrients, in excess of what the body needs, will not do anything to promote the growth of muscle fibers. The growth machinery within the cell must begin first. Muscle stimulation MUST always precede nutrition. If muscular growth is stimulated by high-intensity exercise, the muscles will grow with almost any reasonable diet.

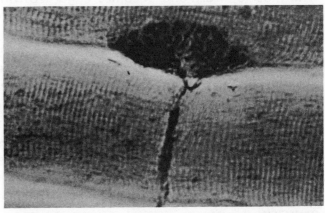
The central nervous system regulates the degree of muscular contraction in a specific movement. This microscopic photograph shows the contact between the nerves and the muscle cells.

The chemical reactions inside growing muscles are much more complicated than exercising and eating. High-intensity muscular contraction results in the formation of a chemical called creatine. The creatine stimulates the muscle to form myosin, one of the contraction proteins within the muscle fiber. Contraction of the muscle fiber produces creatine which causes the muscle to form more myosin. The myosin enables it to undergo more contractions. This causes the production of more creatine which begins the process again.

Creatine has been identified as the messenger substance that turns on the RNA (ribonucleic acid) processing line to produce muscle growth. The RNA within a specialized compartment of the cell acts like an assembly line and hooks together various combinations of amino acids. Those result in the increased size of certain muscle cells. It is important to remember that: First, growth is stimulated through high-intensity exercise. Second, the proper nutrients must be provided for growth.

Q. What is the significance of the tingling in the arms after a hard body-shaping workout?
A. Some women may eventually reach a very high degree of conditioning. This may enable them to exercise their arms intensely. High-intensity body shaping works a maximum percentage of a muscle's fibers and increases demand for nutrient

import and waste export. This is accomplished by elevated blood volume to and from the muscle. The muscle swells and becomes engorged with intercellular fluid.

This engorgement of the arm muscles may produce a dull aching pain. The swelling muscle slightly impinges upon the nerves of the arm, producing a tingling sensation. This sensation is only temporary. Ten minutes or so after termination of the exercise, the aching dissipates as the engorgement diminishes. If a woman is conditioned progressively, this tingling should not be feared. It is indicative of highly effective exercise.

Q. What can a woman do to reduce the large fatty deposits on the sides of her upper thighs?
A. It is impossible to reduce one spot of the body without reducing the whole body. The basic body-shaping and dietary programs recommended in this book will eventually solve the upper thigh problem as the total body is reduced.

Q. What can be done to prevent breast shrinkage during a fat-reduction program?
A. The breasts are largely made up of fat and possess no voluntary muscle. Since a fat-loss program burns fat throughout the body, the breast may become smaller also. Breast shape and contour, however, will improve if the supporting muscular layer beneath them is properly strengthened.

Q. Why should a woman refrain from eating just before exercise?
A. When a woman's large skeletal muscles are activated during strenuous exercise, they require a rich blood supply that provides nutrients and removes waste products. To do this the blood supply to the stomach and intestinal tract is reduced as the blood is mobilized to the working muscles. If food is in the stomach at this time, vomiting may result. It is best not to have eaten a meal within the previous two hours.

Q. Is it true that some foods act as a catalyst to burn other foods?
A. Kelp, apple cider, grapefruit, B6, and lecithin

are some of the products reputed to burn fat. This claim is not true. It is directly opposed to the laws of thermodynamics.

Q. Is it possible to raise the basal metabolism to burn more fat?
A. Basal metabolism is the calories used at rest under laboratory conditions. Most of these calories are related to muscle mass. Stronger, shapelier muscles require more calories than weak, flaccid muscles. Fat cells are inactive. They have fewer blood vessels than muscles have. As a woman grows older her muscles tend to shrink. One reason for this is the failure to maintain physical activity of the type that strengthens the large muscles. A proper fat-loss program, therefore, must include body-shaping and strengthening programs such as those explained in this book.

Q. Is it permissible to skip a meal occasionally?
A. No. Many women who do skip meals have the tendency to nibble later or to overeat at the next meal. They actually end by consuming more calories for the day.

Q. What is more fattening: one high-calorie dessert or the same caloric consumption spread out over a whole day in a number of servings?
A. A calorie is a unit of heat energy. It is the only common denominator for measuring the energy value of fats, proteins, and carbohydrates. During any 24-hour period, a calorie equals another calorie regardless of its source and regardless of whether is is consumed in-part or in-whole.

Q. In relation to losing fat, does the time of day affect the amount of food eaten?
A. It is the total number of calories in a several day period that determines fat loss, not the time of the day, the composition of the food, or the amount.

Q. Why is it so important to count calories instead of carbohydrates?
A. Women sometimes achieve fat reduction utilizing a low-carbohydrate diet. A low-carbohydrate diet is often a low-calorie diet.

The fallacy here is the fact that carbohydrates are only one of the body's three sources of energy. Counting only carbohydrates ignores the possibility of consuming too many calories in the form of fats and proteins.

Also caloric reduction is best achieved by limiting all food consumption, not just one food or class of foods. A low-carbohydrate diet often promotes the ingestion of high quantities of fats, which is undesirable for women with a family history of heart disease.

Q. What is the best way to measure servings of different foods?
A. Servings of food are best measured with a small inexpensive scale, like a postage scale. It is quite accurate for small amounts of food. Volume measures such as cups, pints, and spoons are another possibility.

Q. How can a woman determine the number of calories her body needs each day?
A. It is possible to determine the number of calories needed each day. But it is an expensive and time consuming procedure. An educated guess is, however, possible by using the exact instructions on the following chart:

ESTIMATING CALORIC REQUIREMENTS

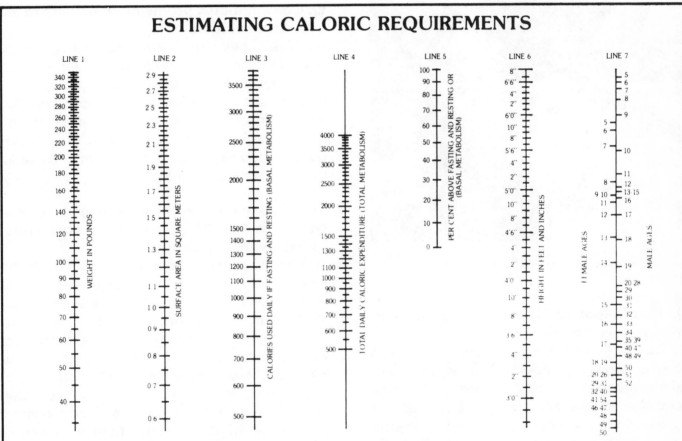

To determine the number of calories you burn in 24 hours, proceed as follows:
1. Using a pin as a marker, locate your actual weight on line 1.
2. Placing the edge of a ruler against the pin, move the other end to your height on line 6.
3. Remove the pin and place it at the point where the ruler crosses line 2.
4. Keeping the edge of the ruler firmly against the pin on line 2, move the right-hand edge to your age and sex on line 7.
5. Remove the pin and place it where the ruler crosses line 3. This gives you the calories used daily if you are resting and fasting.

6. To the basal calories thus determined, add the percentage above fasting and resting for your type of activity or lifestyle. For example, add 50 to 60 percent for manual laborers, active students, and athletes; 30 to 40 percent for typical Americans who participate in nothing more than light work; or 10 to 20 percent for people confined mostly to sitting activities. Leaving the pin in line 3, move the edge of the ruler to the right to the proper percentage on line 5. Where the ruler crosses line 4, you'll find the number of calories necessary to **maintain** your present weight.

FINAL TOUCHES: QUESTIONS AND ANSWERS

Q. How can a woman count calories when eating out?

A. Even when eating out, women must count calories. This becomes a little more difficult than the food measurements that can be performed at home. After a woman acquires some experience at home, however, she will quickly learn to estimate food quantities and their caloric values. This is an indispensable asset when eating out.

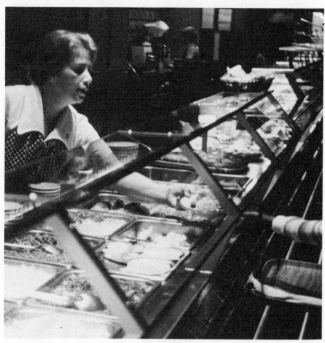

A cafeteria is an inexpensive place to get nutritious food. A weight-conscious woman will select one small serving from each of the four basic food groups.

Q. How important is vitamin supplementation during dieting?

A. The diets recommended in this book have all been designed to provide well-balanced, low-calorie nutrition for most women. The female body has certain self-regulating mechanisms with it and will not use nutrients that are not needed. Considerable money is wasted by taking vitamin pills that the body does not need. If a woman does need vitamin supplementation, her exceptional condition should be evaluated and diagnosed by her physician. Then, only her physician should prescribe what vitamins and dosages are required.

Q. If a woman remains fat even though she thinks that she is eating little in the first place, how can she be helped?

A. Some women have extremely low metabolic rates. This comes from unexplained hereditary factors. Such women can maintain or even accumulate fat on low-calorie intakes. These women possess very efficient metabolisms and must consume even fewer calories in order to lose from their body-fat stores. Such very low-calorie diets probably require a physician's management. Many women who claim to fit into this description, however, actually nibble as they cook or do housework throughout the day. They are not conscious of the amount of food they eat. These women must learn to be more conscious of their eating habits. Keeping a daily dietary diary may be the answer.

Q. Can emotional problems contribute to an over-fat condition?

A. Yes. These problems may range from occasional nervous tension to deep-seated disturbances. A woman may react in two ways to tension: she may either eat or stop eating. An interesting phenomenon is that lean people of normal weight are usually those who, when under tension, stop eating, while their fatter peers tend to stuff themselves under tension.

Q. If a glandular problem is diagnosed in a woman, is it possible that this will contribute to her over-fat condition?

A. The secretions of different glands in the body can affect growth, even fatty growth. A malfunction of these sensitive organs may result in a tendency for a woman to be fat, but she must realize that the resulting fat stores cannot be accumulated without energy-conditioning foodstuff. Her glandular malfunction simply allows her to make extremely efficient use of the foods she eats. If she does not eat those foods, or eats fewer of those foods than an amount necessary to run the body's machinery, fat-loss should still result. For details on glandular conditions, consult a physician.

Q. What about the use of diuretics in a fat-loss program?

A. The use of diuretics as a part of a woman's fat-loss program is strongly discouraged. Diuretics are chemical substances that rid the body of excessive water. A woman must remember, however, that there is very little water in fat. The weight lost from diuretics is not from fatty deposits.

Women who self-administer diuretics may deplete themselves of potassium and other substances. If too much potassium is lost, blood pressure may drop adversely, and serious problems can occur. In addition, the overuse of diuretics can irritate the kidneys, or even lead to diabetes.

Q. How can a woman know whether she is losing weight from loss of fat or from loss of muscle?

A. One easy method to determine the source of bodyweight loss from fat or from muscle is to keep a weekly record of the difference between the relaxed and contracted arm measurements. A woman who is lean and muscular will usually have a difference in these measurements of from ½ to 1 inch. The difference in the relaxed and contracted arm measurements should grow larger as a woman gets leaner. A woman who is carrying too much fat on her body will have little difference in these two measurements.

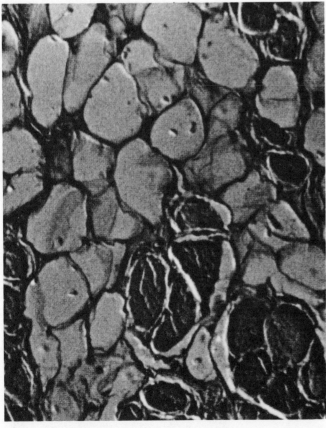

The two most changeable components of a woman's body are fat and muscle. Here both are seen in the same photograph. The fat cells are light colored and the muscle cells are dark. A well-balanced low-calorie diet causes the fat cells to shrink, while proper body shaping demands that the muscle cells get stronger. This combined effect produces more solid and slender flesh.

Q. Women often worry about water retention just before their period. How should they interpret their bodyweight fluctuations due to this phenomenon?

A. A woman must realize that a fat-loss program is exactly that -- a fat-loss program, not a water-loss program. If she continues to lose fat with a low-calorie dietary plan, but retains water for a few days, the scales may show increased bodyweight. Weight may not always show a reduction of fat, especially when water retention is concerned. Fat contains very little water.

Q. Why does bodyweight suddenly plateau after a woman has faithfully followed her reduction program for a week or so?

A. Certain women tend to retain fluid as they lose fat. Even though they are losing fat, it does not show on the scale, at least not for several weeks. This plateau is usually a temporary phenomenon, and after a few weeks, these women will once again begin to lose weight on a low-calorie diet.

Q. Are there any "crutches" to help a woman as she adjusts to a reducing diet?

A. Here are a few harmless actions a woman can take to obtain oral gratification at low-calorie costs:
1. Chew sugarless gum
2. Drink ice water
3. Drink diet soda
4. Munch on a carrot or celery stick
5. Go for a walk
6. Do some vigorous exercise
7. Call a friend on the phone

Q. How often should a woman weigh herself when on a fat-reduction diet?

A. Even though women may register a few unexplained gains, there is merit in weighing every day and plotting the weight on a chart. Some women tend to retain water for a while during weight loss. Most pre-menopausal women retain some water every month before menstruation.

Q. If fad diets are so ineffective, why do many woman subscribe to them?

A. Fad diets are popular among women today primarily for two reasons:

FINAL TOUCHES: QUESTIONS AND ANSWERS

1. The widespread ignorance of proper nutritional and dietary principles among women.
2. A natural tendency for all people to accept the easiest answer to their personal problems.

Q. How long does a woman need to continue this body-shaping, fat-reducing program?
A. A woman who successfully applies the principles of this program will want to continue it for the rest of her life.

Losing fat and keeping it off permanently is a life-long commitment to proper body shaping and well-balanced, low-calorie eating.

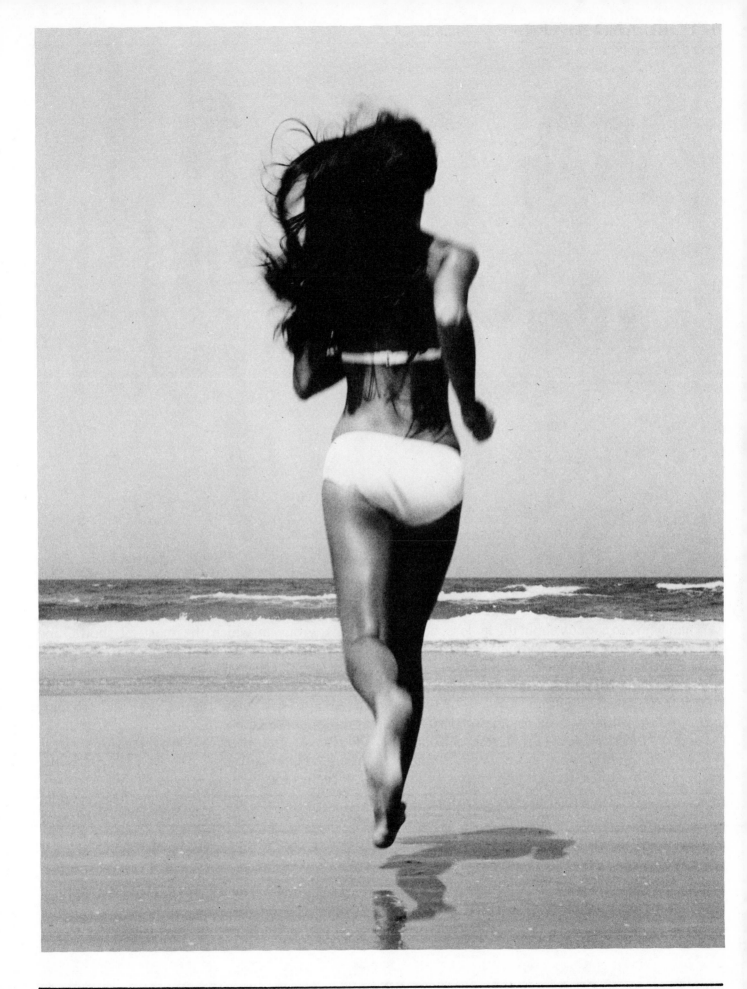

FINAL TOUCHES: QUESTIONS AND ANSWERS

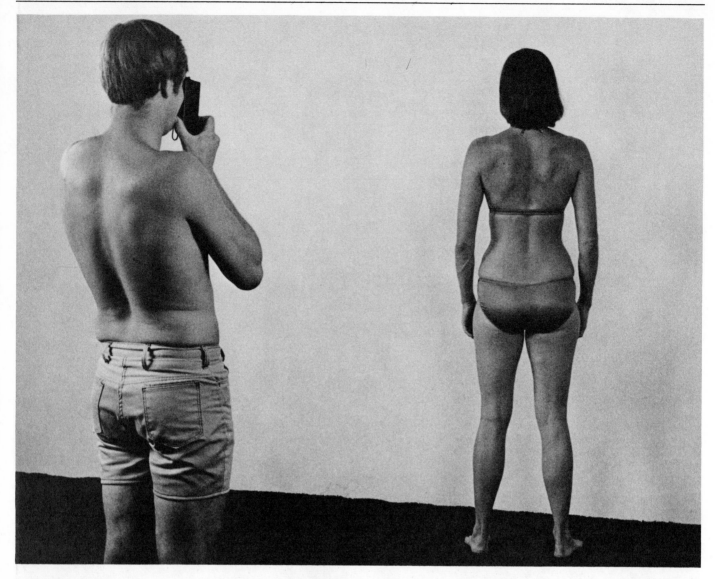

Women who are serious about the fat-loss, body-shaping program can have a visual record of their progress by following these directions:
• Wear a snug bathing suit and have full-length photographs taken against an uncluttered background. Do not try to pose. Stand perfectly relaxed for three pictures — front, side, and back.
• Have two prints of each negative made. On the back of each photograph in both sets write the date and bodyweight. File one set for safe keeping.
• Select the worst photograph of the remaining set, the one in which the most fat shows, and carry it around in a billfold or pocketbook. Look at it often, especially before meals and before retiring.
• Adhere strictly to the fat-loss, body-shaping program in this book.
• Repeat the picture-taking sessions every month. Compare the photographs with the preceding sets.
• Use the before-and-after pictures as a reminder of the previous state of fatness and as motivation for continued fat loss and body shaping.

CONCLUSION

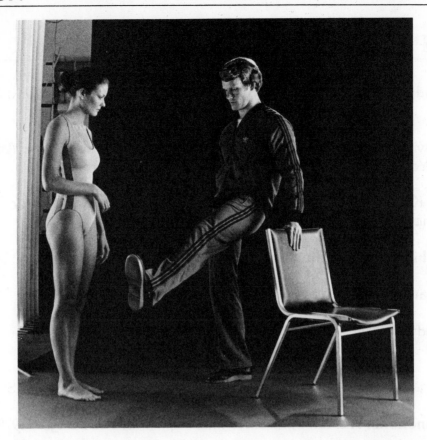

From fatness to fitness is not an easy road to travel. Many turn back along the way. But those who discipline themselves to travel it consistently will reach their goal of a beautiful, slender, shapely body.

The signposts along the road are clearly marked in this book:

Exercise slowly.
Exercise strenuously.
Exercise briefly.
Eat nutritiously
Eat moderately.
Reshape permanently.

Dr. Ellington Darden is an authority in the field of physical fitness, body shaping, and nutrition. He holds B.S. and M.S. degrees from Baylor University, a Ph.D. from Florida State University, and has had two years of post-doctoral study in food and nutrition. He is a well-known writer and speaker whose books, articles, and lectures are bringing a new awareness of body fitness to Americans of all ages.

As Director of Research for Nautilus Sports/Medical Industries, he has trained numerous college and professional athletes as well as many middle-aged men and women.

In the photograph above Dr. Darden is explaining the one-legged squat to Lona Dion. Lona and her husband Ken own and operate several Nautilus fitness centers in the Philadelphia area. Scott LeGear's photographs of Lona's shapely body appear throughout this book.

BIBLIOGRAPHY

Astrand, Per-Olof, and Rodahl, Kaare. **Textbook of Work Physiology.** New York: McGraw-Hill Book Co., 1977.

Baron, Howard C., with Gorin, Edward. **Varicose Veins: A Commonsense Approach to Their Management.** New York: William Morrow & Co., 1979.

Barrett, Stephen, and Knight, Gilda (editors). **The Health Robbers: How to Protect Your Money and Your Life.** Philadelphia: George F. Stickley Co., Publishers, 1976.

Bayrd, Edwin. **The Thin Game: Dieting Scams and Dietary Sense.** New York: Avon Books, 1979.

Beller, Anne Scott. **Fat and Thin.** New York: Farrar, Straus and Giroux, 1977.

Briggs, George M., and Calloway, Doris H. **Bogert's Nutrition and Physical Fitness.** Philadelphia: W.B. Saunders Co., 1979.

Consumer Guide Magazine. **The Complete Guide to Building a Better Body.** Stokie, Illinois, 1979.

Crouch, James E. **Functional Human Anatomy.** Philadelphia: Lea & Febiger, 1978.

Darden, Ellington. **Nutrition for Athletes: Myths and Truths.** Winter Park, Florida: Anna Publishing, Inc., 1978.

Darden, Ellington. **How Your Muscles Work.** Winter Park, Florida: Anna Publishing, Inc. 1978.

Darden, Ellington. **Strength-Training Principles.** Winter Park, Florida: Anna Publishing, Inc. 1977.

Darden, Ellington, "What Research Says About Positive and Negative Work," **Scholastic Coach** 45: 6, 7, October 1975.

"Delusions of Vigor: Better Health by Mail," **Consumer Reports** 44: 50-54, January, 1979.

Deutsch, Ronald M. **The New Nuts Among the Berries.** Palo Alto, California: Bull Publishing Co., 1977.

Edington, D.W., and Edgerton, V.R. **The Biology of Physical Activity.** Boston: Houghton Mifflin Co., 1976.

Hirsch, Jules, and Knittle, Jerome L. "Cellularity of Obese and Non-obese Human Adipose Tissue," **Federation Proceedings** 29: 1516-1521, 1970.

Howe, Phyllis S. **Basic Nutrition in Health and Disease.** Philadelphia: W.B. Saunders Co., 1976.

Jones, Arthur. "Negative Work as a Factor in Exercise," **Athletic Journal** 55: 54, 60, 86, April 1975.

Jones, Arthur. "Progressive Exercise: Intensity and Strength," **Athletic Journal** 55: 76-69, September, 1974.

Jones, Arthur. **Nautilus Training Principles, Bulletins #1 and 2.** Deland, Florida: Nautilus Sports/Medical Industries, 1970.

Katch, Frank I., and McArdle, William D. **Nutrition, Weight Control, and Exercise.** Boston: Houghton Mifflin Co., 1977.

Lamb, David R. **Physiology of Exercise: Responses and Adaptations.** New York: Macmillan Publishing Co., Inc., 1978.

Mathews, Donald K., and Fox, Edward L. **The Physiological Basis of Physical Education and Athletics.** Philadelphia: W.B. Saunders Co., 1976.

Melnick, Daniel. **A Teaching Manual on Food and Nutrition for Non-Science Majors.** Washington, D.C.: The Nutrition Foundation, Inc., 1979.

McNutt, Kristen, and McNutt, David R. **Nutrition and Food Choices.** Chicago: Science Research Associates, Inc., 1978.

Oglesby, Carole A. **Woman and Sport: From Myth to Reality.** Philadelphia: Lea & Febiger, 1978.

Peterson, James A. (editor). **Conditioning for a Purpose: How to Become Physically Fit for Sports and Athletes.** West Point, New York: Leisure Press, 1977.

Rasch, Philip J., and Burke, Roger K. **Kinesiology and Applied Anatomy.** Philadelphia: Lea & Febiger, 1978.

Rivenes, Richard S. **Foundations of Physical Education.** Boston: Houghton Mifflin Co., 1978.